Sponsored by the
European Association of Neurosurgical Societies

Advances and Technical Standards in Neurosurgery

Edited by

L. Symon, London (Editor-in-Chief)
L. Calliauw, Gent
F. Cohadon, Bordeaux
J. Lobo Antunes, Lisbon
F. Loew, Homburg/Saar
H. Nornes, Oslo
E. Pásztor, Budapest
J. D. Pickard, Southampton
A. J. Strong, London
M. G. Yaşargil, Zurich

Volume 18

Springer-Verlag Wien GmbH

With 27 Figures

Originally published by Springer-Verlag/Wien in 1991

Library of Congress Catalog Card Number 74-10499

ISSN 0095-4829

ISBN 978-3-7091-7385-5 ISBN 978-3-7091-6697-0 (eBook)

DOI 10.1007/978-3-7091-6697-0

The Decade of the Brain

In many countries, principally under the stimulation of the United States, the 1990 s have been declared the decade of the brain.

Although a great deal of progress has been made in neurological and neurosurgical research in the past hundred years, neurological disease remains a major contributor to disability and death throughout the world. With the increasing age of the population in the developed countries problems of stroke and neuronal degeneration play an increasing part in determining the pattern of health care in the aged, and a great deal of national resource becomes devoted to the management of conditions which may be preventable.

Many new powerful techniques of clinical research are available, magnetic resonance spectroscopy, magnetic resonance imaging, positron tomography and genetic analysis all require funding to an extent which demands governmental assistance.

The editors welcome the concept of the "decade of the brain". Neuroscientists in both clinic and laboratory are anxious to press forward their understanding of the pathophysiology of major brain disease and to advance the philosophy of brain protection and prevention of disability. Much has been done, much is within our grasp but all requires not only the efforts of dedicated scientists but extensive government funding. We look forward to practical results of this initiative and wish it well.

The Editors

Preface

As an addition to the European postgraduate training system for young neurosurgeons we began to publish in 1974 this series devoted to Advances and Technical Standards in Neurosurgery which was later sponsored by the European Association of Neurosurgical Societies.

The fact that the English language is well on the way to becoming the international medium at European scientific conferences is a great asset in terms of mutual understanding. Therefore we have decided to publish all contributions in English, regardless of the native language of the authors.

All contributions are submitted to the entire editorial board before publication of any volume.

Our series is not intended to compete with the publications of original scientific papers in other neurosurgical journals. Our intention is, rather, to present fields of neurosurgery and related areas in which important recent advances have been made. The contributions are written by specialists in the given fields and constitute the first part of each volume.

In the second part of each volume, we publish detailed descriptions of standard operative procedures, furnished by experienced clinicians; in these articles the authors describe the techniques they employ and explain the advantages, difficulties and risks involved in the various procedures. This part is intended primarily to assist young neurosurgeons in their postgraduate training. However, we are convinced that it will also be useful to experienced, fully trained neurosurgeons.

The descriptions of standard operative procedures are a novel feature of our series. We intend that this section should make available the findings of European neurosurgeons, published perhaps in less familiar languages, to neurosurgeons beyond the boundaries of the authors countries and of Europe. We will however from time to time bring to the notice of our European colleagues, operative procedures from colleagues in the United States and Japan, who have developed techniques which may now be regarded as standard. Our aim throughout is to promote contacts among neurosurgeons in Europe and throughout the world neurosurgical community in general.

We hope therefore that surgeons not only in Europe, but throughout the world will profit by this series of Advances and Technical Standards in Neurosurgery.

The Editors

Contents

Listed in Index Medicus

A. Advances

B. Technical Standards

List of Contributors

Adamson, Dr. T. E., Neurochirurgische Klinik, Universitätsspital Zürich, Rämistraße 100, CH-8091 Zürich, Switzerland.

Bastide, Dr. R., Clinique Universitaire de Neurochirurgie, CHU Toulouse Rangueil, Avenue J. Poulhès, F-31054 Toulouse Cedex, France.

Benabid, Prof. Dr. A. L., Head of Neurosurgery, Director of INSERM U 318, Grenoble University Hospital, BP 217X, F-38043 Grenoble, France.

Castel, Dr. J. P., Clinique Universitaire de Neurochirurgie, Groupe Hospitalier Pellegrin, Place A. Raba Léon, F-33076 Bordeaux, France.

Cinquin, Prof. Dr. Ph., UFR of Medicine, Grenoble University Hospital, BP 217X, F-38043 Grenoble, France.

Danel, Dr. F., 21 Avenue Jeanne d'Arc, F-38100 Grenoble, France.

Demongeot, Prof. Dr. J., Head of Biomathematics, UFR of Medicine, Grenoble University Hospital, BP 217X, F-38043 Grenoble, France.

Dietz, Prof. Dr. H., Direktor der Neurochirurgischen Klinik der Medizinischen Hochschule Hannover, Karl-Wiechert-Allee, D-W-3000 Hannover 61 (Kleefeld) Federal Republic of Germany.

Hoffmann, Dr. D., Department of Neurosurgery, Grenoble University Hospital, BP 217X, F-38043 Grenoble, France.

Lavallée, Dr. S., UFR of Medicine, Grenoble University Hospital, BP 217X, Grenoble, France.

Lazorthes, Prof. Dr. Y., Clinique Universitaire de Neurochirurgie, CHU Toulouse-Rangueil, Avenue J. Poulhès, F-31054 Toulouse Cedex, France.

Le Bas, Prof. Dr. J.-F., Head of MRI, Grenoble University Hospital, BP 217X, F-38043 Grenoble, France.

Roth, Dr. P., Neurochirurgische Klinik, Universitätsspital Zürich, Rämistraße 100, CH-8091 Zürich, Switzerland.

Sallerin-Caute, Dr. B., Clinique Universitaire de Neurochirurgie, CHU Toulouse-Rangueil, Avenue J. Poulhès, F-31054 Toulouse Cedex, France.

Tranmer, Dr. B. I., Neurochirurgische Klinik, Universitätsspital Zürich, Rämistraße 100, CH-8091 Zürich, Switzerland.

Verdie, Dr. J. C., Clinique Universitaire de Neurochirurgie, CHU Toulouse-Rangueil, Avenue J. Poulhès, F-31054 Toulouse Cedex, France.

Yaşargil, Prof. Dr. M. G., Neurochirurgische Klinik, Universitätsspital Zürich, Rämistraße 100, CH-8091 Zürich, Switzerland.

A. Advances

Is There any Future for Robots in Neurosurgery?

A. L. Benabid[1, 3], D. Hoffmann[1, 3], S. Lavallee[2], P. Cinquin[2], J. Demongeot[2], J. F. Le Bas[1, 4], and F. Danel

[1] Unité INSERM U. 318, Neurobiologie Préclinique, Laboratoire de Neurobiophysique, UFR de Médecine, Université Joseph Fourier de Grenoble
[2] Laboratoire de Biomathématiques, UFR de Médecine, Université Joseph Fourier de Grenoble
[3] Service de Neurochirurgie
[4] Unité d'Imagerie par Résonance Magnétique

CHU Albert Michallon, Grenoble (France)

With 11 Figures

Contents

I. Introduction

Since the first conception of machines that could replace humans for tasks they used to perform, the development of increasingly intelligent machines, later called robots, led to the science of synnoetics[1] implying the perfect integration of humans and robots in an harmonious society. Science-fiction literature has helped us grow accustomed to the idea and the theme of mankind threatened by dominating robotic creatures has rapidly gone out of style. The prospect of an increasingly robotized society is becoming more acceptable and the recent experience of robots entering the exclusive domain of medicine has proven that they are regarded as an addition to skill and safety rather than as a danger. Incredibly rapid progress in computer science, artificial intelligence, biomedical engineering and medical imaging, together with our society's never ending pursuit of higher medical standards and achievements will undoubtedly foster advancements in medical robotics far beyond the scope of present-day capabilities. However, before a time has come when intelligent and flexible robots will be able to integrate the sum of clinical and paraclinical data, state a diagnosis, make a decision, and then perform a therapeutic (including surgical) procedure, not in a completely pre-programmed but in an adaptative manner based on the immediate knowledge provided by their own sensors, a considerable amount of work remains to be done well beyond the current state of the art. It is without doubt that the feed-back loop between the potential commercial market, industrial creativity and efficiency, and the subsequent new applications in medicine will accelerate this process. For the time-being, to remain objective, we can only review whence we came and where we are to-day.

The particular susceptibility of nervous tissue in the brain, has naturally tended to minimize the trauma of neurosurgical procedures including surgical approaches. This attitude culminates in the "keyhole neurosurgery" concept, which imposes two complementary prerequisites: precision of target and narrowness of approach. The second has been made possible by technical advances in endoscopy, fiber optics, microinstrumentation and the use of physical agents capable of being transported along thin pathways (such as heat and laser). The first prerequisite has been addressed for several years now by such methods as stereotaxy[7, 20, 67–69, 71–74]. The increasing application of stereotaxy, the availability of sophisticated and predigitized imaging modalities (CT-scan, MRI, DSA, US imaging) and the expanding power of computers call for integration of these technical opportunities[21, 49, 53, 54, 79]. Robotization of neurosurgical procedures is the logical and mandatory consequence of these developments. This was already recognized several years ago by P. Kelly[23, 28–41] and, later by R. Young[80] and Y. S. Kwoh[43–45]. What remains to be accomplished, as well as the work presented here, is nothing more than the development of their original and pioneering ideas.

II. Robotics in Medicine and Neurosurgery: History and General Principles

II.1 History of the Robotics Concept in Medicine

Although robotization can be foreseen in a wide range of medical and surgical procedures, current applications mainly concern stereotaxy. Computerization and robotization are inherently present in the basic principle of stereotaxy. This principle encompasses a natural evolution towards precision, repetition, automation of parts or even to entire procedures, automatic adaptation of procedures to specific, anatomic parameters of the patient, report of procedure parameters to control data bases such as anatomic atlases, and interactivity and feed back processes between the databases and the current procedure. The history of stereotaxy[20] is already rich in examples of such attempts of motorization, automation, and even computerization. Indeed, the present burst of computer and information technology has boosted this original tendency[40] and made concrete what was some years ago no more than a science fiction cartoon. Atlas computerization was first reported at the Edinburgh meeting of the Society for Stereotaxy and Functional Neurosurgery, in 1972. Later computerization of stereotactic calculation was attempted or achieved through CT-adapted stereotaxy[12, 16, 21, 23, 29, 38, 49, 53], and in 1982 P. Kelly[36] described the first routine application of computer assisted neurosurgery, confirming the potential future for such an approach. In the 1990's this concept will undoubtedly come to maturity and extend widely to the general field of computer assisted medicosurgical procedures. Current problems concerning ethics and safety, already brought to public attention[1], have to be kept in mind and resolved.

II.2 General Principles of a Neurosurgical Robotized Set-up (Fig. 1)

At the present time, all robotized neurosurgical procedures involve stereotactic frames, which provide fixation of the head and, therefore, a stable position of the brain in the robot space, after calibration is done. It is expected that technical progress will show the performance of at least some neurosurgical procedures without holding the head firmly in a frame, provided that the head position can be monitored during surgery with a precision high enough to be compatible with the degree of precision required by the involved procedure. Currently, a regular set-up consists of a robot linked to a frame, the varying relationships of which are checked using an X-ray system. There are some specific considerations regarding the integration of frames and X-ray systems with the robotized system.

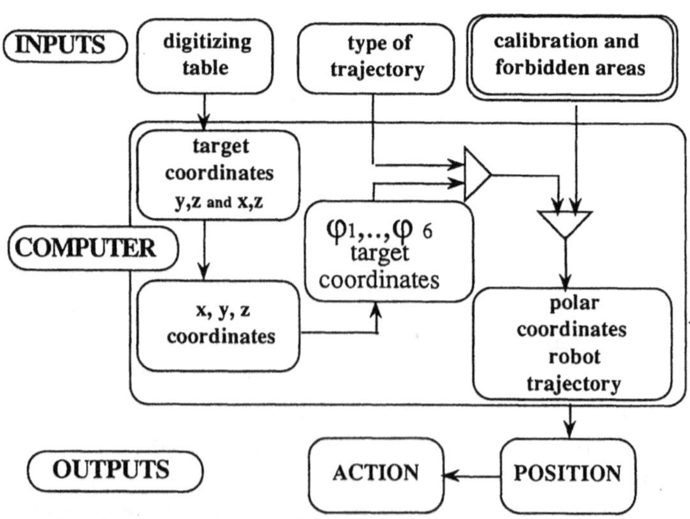

Fig. 1. General diagram of a robot system and flow chart of the software

A. Stereotactic Frames

A stereotactic frame is essentially used to hold the head in a stable position with respect to the robot. Therefore, all types of frames would be acceptable as long as they are rigid and have few external features in order to limit the risk of collisions with the robot. Compatibility of frames with CT-scanners and MRI systems must be considered, as well as reproducibility of patient placement, and flexibility of the frame which must have detachable parts in order to move the patient from the robot set-up to other operating rooms. It is generally admitted that stereotaxy was invented in 1905 by Horsley and Clarke[26] who needed an accurate tool for electrode insertion and lesion making in laboratory animals. This laboratory equipment was later adapted for neurosurgical purposes by Spiegel and Wycis in 1947[64] although the first human stereotactic apparatus was probably built in London around 1919 by Aubrey Mussen who had worked with Clarke[55]. This made functional surgery possible at the level of deep brain structures such as the basal ganglia and third ventricle. The introduction of pallido-thalamotomy following the accidental observation of Cooper led to considerable development in stereotaxy as a conventional neurosurgical procedure. The evident need for accuracy, reproducibility, safety, and minimized invasiveness is responsible for the design of several types of stereotactic frames, each of them addressing a specific concern. Logically enough, the majority of frames during the first half of the century were mainly designed for procedures involving stereotactic lesions on the basal ganglia, which represented the only surgical treatment of Parkinson's disease and of other types of dyskinesias. The apparently unappealing aspect of calculating target coordinates restricted stereotaxy to a narrow set of "mathematically - minded" neurosurgeons. The recent possibility of linking stereotactic frames and CT-scanners, with adequate software to calculate target coordinates and frame parameter values required before surgery, has made this procedure available to a larger group of neurosurgeons. Although this constitutes a real improvement, this newly available simplicity has contributed to a tremendous increase in the practice of stereotactic neurosurgery and possibly to an increased risk of haemorrhagic complications. All stereotactic frames share a common purpose which is to establish rigid relationships between the patient's head and brain, and the outer space which contains surgical tools, such as cannulae, probes, electrodes, or larger systems such as X-ray tubes used either for neuroradiological examination or for radiosurgery. All frames are always firmly anchored to the patient's skull by several pins, (at least 3 and usually 4) more or less deeply inserted into the bone. Less invasive relationships, such as fixation by ear plugs and nose and neck positioners, have been used, but are not compatible with precise and stable positioning.

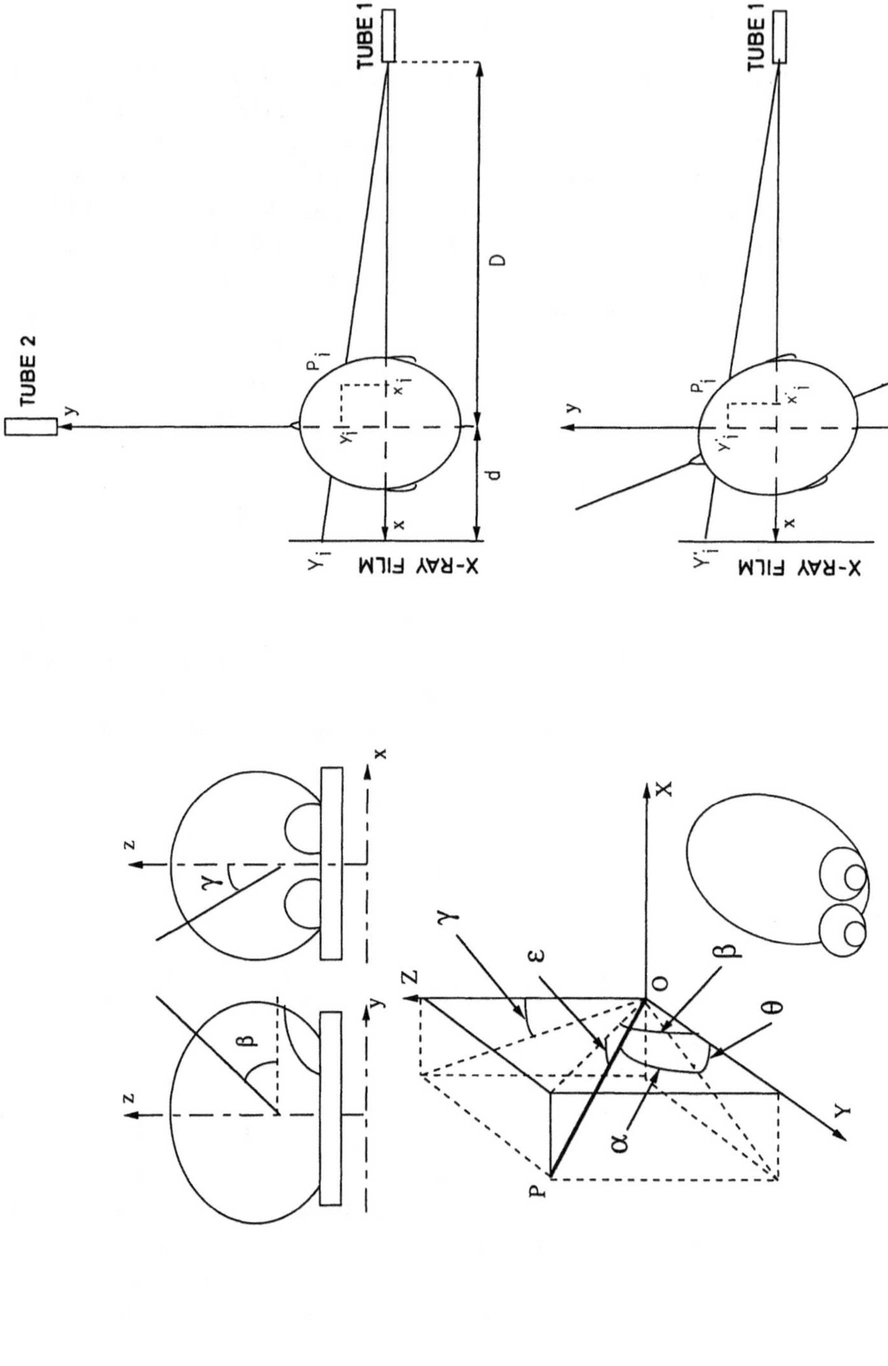

Fig. 2. Cartesian and spherical coordinates of a given point P

Two main types of frames can be considered, depending on how the target is reached: the first type, which comprises the Leksell-Elekta, Riechert-Mundinger-Fischer, OBT and similar frames, is mainly based on a center-of-arch system allowing double oblique trajectories aimed at central targets. Their relatively small size has allowed them to be redesigned with X-ray transparent and amagnetic materials, making them compatible with CT-scan and MRI systems. The visibility of the frame structures and fiducial markers on these imaging systems has been used to develop software providing easy calculation of the coordinates to be set up on the frame in order to reach a given target designated on CT-scan or MRI pictures. In the Leksell-type frames, an arch-goniometer is designed to reach the center of the arch with special (fixed-length) probes. The center of the arch can be projected onto X-ray films and precisely placed in front of the antero-posterior and lateral projections of the target by displacements of the arch support on the frame. In other cases, (Mundinger-Riechert) arch system parameters are determined using a specific paradigm and are checked on a phantom. The development of computer software adapted to CT-scan and MRI examination has more recently provided the possibility to determine easily the coordinates and characteristics of the tracks, in biorthogonal or double-oblique approaches, from the target as visible on the image display. This is particularly convenient when the target is clearly defined, which is the case for brain tumours, the size of which is larger than the accuracy of the pixel size of the images.

The second type, represented by the Talairach frame[71–74] is mainly based on orthogonal (frontal or lateral) approaches. The Talairach frame essentially features a rectangular base with four pilars supporting calibrated screws holding the fixation pins, a system of double grids (allowing orthogonal tool penetration into the brain along directions parallel to the X-ray beams) and added sets to accessories: the Sedan[61] and Scerratti[58] goniometers have been conceived and designed to provide the Talairach system with the advantages and flexibility of the center-of-arch systems allowing easy and precise access via oblique approaches to targets near the midline. Correspondance between the x, y, z cartesian coordinates of a point P, the α and θ angles of the ρ, α, θ spherical coordinates, the β and γ angles read on the X-rays, and the β and ε angles set up on the goniometer are given by the following simple equations (Fig. 2):

$$
\begin{aligned}
\rho &= OP \\
x &= \rho \cdot \cos\alpha \cdot \sin\theta \\
y &= \rho \cdot \cos\alpha \cdot \cos\theta \\
z &= \rho \cdot \sin\alpha \\
\beta &= \text{Arctan}\ (\tan\alpha/\cos\theta) \\
\gamma &= \text{Arctan}\ (\sin\theta/\tan\alpha) \\
\varepsilon &= \text{Arctan}\ (x/(x^2 + z^2)^{1/2})
\end{aligned}
$$

Whatever the type of robot used, the system should fulfill the following prerequisites:

– reproducible patient placement: this can be achieved by a heavy frame base, which cannot be distorted by current mechanical stresses, and by four strong pins which are inserted into burr holes drilled through the full depth of the skull, held by verniers the graduations of which are recorded and can be replicated.

– perfect orthogonality of the X-ray beams in the antero-posterior and lateral directions: this can be achieved by a specific set-up in the operating room, and by repeated control of correct placement of the frame at the focus point of the X-ray set-up.

– precise knowledge of the central X-ray beam, either placed on the area of interest, centered on the target, or used for exact correction of the parallax distortion due to a beam centered at distance from the target.

– superimposition of modalities:

The pins inserted into the skull are in a fixed and reproducible position and their appearance is the same on every X-ray picture, taken during the same or different stereotactic sessions, provided that the pin holding verniers are each time set at identical values. Therefore, matching the pin projections on the X-ray pictures, provides the possibility of superimposing different modalities, (such as angiograms, ventriculograms, or any other kind of image acquired in stereotactic conditions) so that a synthetic diagram can be drawn.

However this system imposes important hindrances which might discourage users and push them towards apparently easier systems, or more dangerously, towards less secure and careful procedures.

The differences between frames are more related to the industrial features than to the methodological principles, since a frame can be likened to a simple pair of "sugar-tongs" holding the skull and the brain in a fixed postion.

B. X-ray Systems

A stereotactic frame must be positioned at the focus of a bi-directional double-tube X-ray system, the beams of which are orthogonal. A first tube is located at the ceiling of the operating room, with its axis in the vertical direction and is used for antero-posterior views of the patient's head in the supine position. The second tube, with its axis in the horizontal direction is located in a side part of the room, for lateral X-ray views of the patient's head. Both tubes are at a long distance from the head, depending on the room set-up, but always greater than 3 meters. This achieves a low magnification ratio which is equal to 1.05 in our set-up where tubes are 3.75 meters away from the center of the frame. This ratio is precisely determined by the respective positions of the tube, the patient's head, and the film. Actually, the magnification ratio is different for each point of the brain, depending on its relative position with respect to the tubes and X-ray film, and involves special computations which are developed below.

The Talairach frame holds two sets of grids placed on the sides of the frame base and which are perpendicular two by two. Making calculation easier and taking maximal advantage of the frame properties requires orthogonality of the grids and of the corresponding X-ray beams. This is achieved by precise positioning of the frame at the beginning of the procedure. This can be accomplished using a laser beam which is coaxial with the X-ray beam and laser reflectors on the frame. Another way consists in mounting the Talairach frame on a solid state base, strongly fixed to the floor of the room, and initially positioned at the center of the X-ray system. In both cases, the X-ray system has to be perfectly perpendicular. As a consequence of this set-up, the altitude Z of a given point in space in the brain with respect to the plane of the frame, which is named the "horizontal" plane of the brain, is the same on the two, antero-posterior (frontal view) and lateral, X-ray pictures. This is very useful to determine whether or not a point in the vascular bed which appears to intersect the track of biopsies actually does. If so, this track must have the same Z values of the projections of its suspected vascular intersection on both frontal and lateral projections, as explained below.

III. State of the Art of Medical Robotics

The current state of medical robotics comprises robots used as therapeutic tools in neurosurgery, and other applications such as in ophthalmology or in nursing care. Work has been reported by other authors in neurosurgical stereotaxy[19] and in diverse medical applications[78] but is still at the laboratory experimental level. To our knowledge, with the exception of Kelly's and our own work, no other experience in routine robotized neurosurgery has thus far been reported. We shall consider the different approaches which are reported at the present time in neurosurgery and other medical fields.

III.1. Robots in Neurosurgery

A. Stereotactic Robots

Three systems aimed at performing the usual stereotactic procedures using robots as a surgical tool are currently in existence.

A.1. The Kwoh-Young (Long Beach) System (Fig. 3)

This system was undoubtedly the first stereotactic robot ever designed and built. It includes a PUMA robot system manufactured by Unimation, Inc.

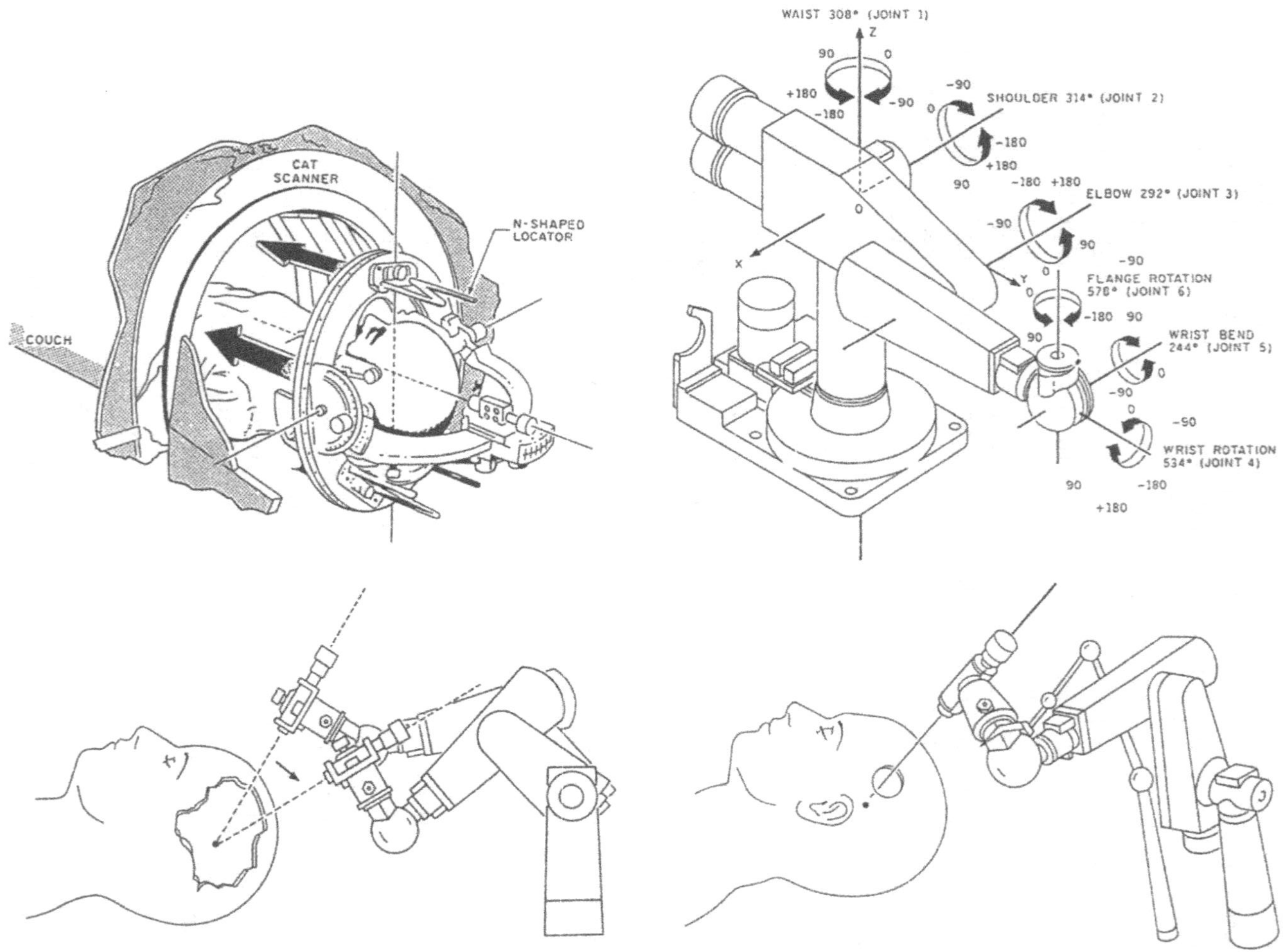

Fig. 3. The Long Beach system: General structure and examples of procedures. (With permission of the authors)

The mechanical arm of the robot has six joints. Each joint is driven by a permanent magnet servomotor through a gear train. The waist, shoulder, and elbow incorporate electromagnetic brakes which are activated when the power is cut off. All servomotors incorporate optical incremental encoders that provide position and velocity feedback to the robot's servo-system. A probe holder is attached to the end effector of the arm. The electronic controller contains a DEC LSI-11 minicomputer as well as digital and analog circuits to control each of the robot's joints and its power supply. A manual control unit allows the user to manipulate the robot through different buttons and a speed-control switch. In case of emergency, all processes can be stopped and every joint of the robot arm is frozen. The LSI-11 computer is designed for robot control only and lacks the software needed for stereotactic computation. A host computer (Data General Eclipse or DEC 11/34) is used to store the CAT-scan images and run the stereotactic software. The head of the patient is held by four stainless steel-tipped screw pins in a stereotactic frame attached to the scanner couch's sliding surface and supports 3 N-shaped locators. The X-Y coordinates of a target selected on an image are transformed into the robot's 3 D coordinate system. The choice of an additional entry point leads to the determination of the trajectory on which the robot probe holder will align itself. The robot arm is used to guide burr hole drilling and to insert the probe, while the robot and effector is locked by clamping it with an external stand. This system is capable of placing probes to a cartesian coordinate precision of 0.05 mm. The designers of the PUMA system recognize that the PUMA 200 may not be the ideal candidate for stereotactic robotized surgery. They emphasize that their intention was to demonstrate the effectiveness of a robot in these procedures and the potential for robotic stereotaxy becoming the core of an integrated computerized system for delicate surgery. Even if their system has not been used routinely in clinical applications, their work was indeed pioneering[43–45, 80].

A.2. The Grenoble Stereotactic Robot System

1. Description of the System

The structure of the Grenoble Robot System is a logical consequence of the needs, difficulties, and frustrations which are experienced during the daily practice of stereotaxy applied to a wide variety of diseases, such as brain tumours, dyskinesias, pain and epilepsy. A list of prerequisites was used to outline the project, in a way similar to the Long Beach project. The system had to be:

– precise and reliable.

– capable of performing every kind of routine stereotactic procedure using the same frame and equipment.

— driven from various types of neuroradiological images (X-Rays, CT-Scan, MRI) from which the target would be defined with accuracy to less than one millimeter.

— safe, and permanently submissive to human control for safety reasons as well as for iterative corrections of the programmed trajectory.

— capable of including sub-routine softwares which could be applied to sophisticated but stereotyped procedures, such as thalamic approaches for thalamotomies or electrode implantations, based on simple radiological landmarks.

— subsequently integrated into a larger system, including if needed, other kinds of neuro-imaging as well as databases such as computer-resident atlases.

— a possible first step towards other therapeutic applications such as multibeam convergent irradiation and computer guided "open neurosurgery". In addition, the project needed to consider the development of user friendly human/computer interfaces, versatility towards future applications, and the maintenance of reasonable costs compatible with conventional hospital practice.

The system described here is as present in daily routine use at the Grenoble University Hospital; it comprises a robot physically linked to a stereotactic frame and driven by a computer according to target coordinates provided by a digitizing table. This basic system can be connected to a digitized angiography system, to the main computer of a MR imager through an Ethernet network, and to a central computer where these images are processed, 3 D pictures are generated and where the stereotactic atlas data are stored.

Till now, the Talairach frame has been used in Grenoble. It consists of a base plate holding four pilars bearing the verniers of the pins. Any other frame can be used provided that exact placement of the patient is possible and that the calibration and definition of forbidden areas, due to the external features of the frame, have been established for this particular frame. The frame is mounted on a rotating ring which allows complete examination of the ventricular system by X-rays in the supine, lateral and recumbent positions. The rotating system is itself mounted on a solid base firmly attached to the floor and to the base of the robot. The center of the frame is situated at the crossing point of the beams of two X-ray tubes permanently positioned at 3.5 meters from the frame, one on the ceiling of the operating room for antero-posterior views, the other on a wall of the room for lateral views.

The robot presently in use is a 6 axis robot, (Fig. 3) derived from a universal industrial robot[3, 8, 9, 46] which has been specially redesigned to match the specific requirements of stereotaxy. Basically, it is designed to be slower, since speed is not necessary, and as precise as possible. Maximal safety, which comes naturally from these two specifications has also been given special attention. The position encoders on each axis have been set up to 200,000 encoding pulses per turn, to achieve a resolution of 360°/200,000 = $1.8\ 10^{-3}$ degree. High reduction gears have been incorporated in order to reduce the maximal speed (about 0.02 turn/sec on each axis), and. most of all, to eliminate the risk of back-driving when the servo-control and the power of the motors are cut off. The dimensions of the various parts of the robot are human-like and allow a comparable spatial field of action, in half a sphere around the head of a patient in the recumbent position. The robot is fixed on a solid base screwed on the floor. It has a trunk, shoulder, arm, elbow, forearm, wrist and hand and all parts are connected by six angular joints. The trunk of the robot, 30 cms high, can turn 270° around its vertical axis. The shoulder, which is at 100 cms above the floor (at the same height as the patient's head), holds the arm, which is 35 cms long and has 180° of liberty. The forearm, 45 cms long, is connected to the arm by the elbow which is allowed to turn over 270°, and is terminated by a wrist, made of 3 combined axes, having respectively 270°, 180° and 270° of freedom for the first, second and third axis. The end plate of the wrist is adaptable to specific tools or "hands", which can be designed for special tasks. At the present time, the fingers of the hand, which perform skills, are limited to a guide tube (Fig. 4), which can be

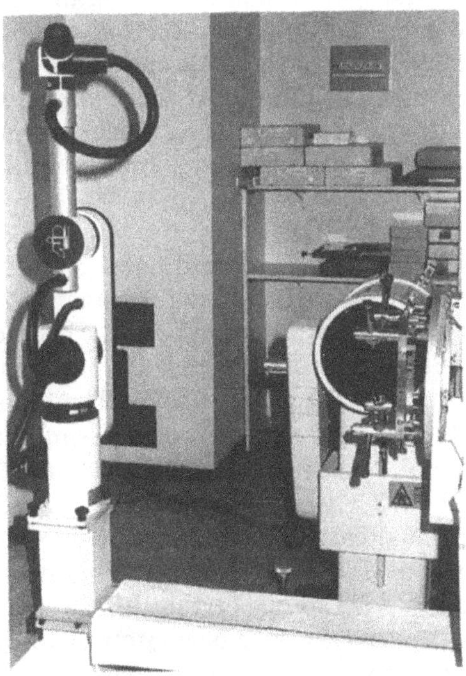

Fig. 4. The Grenoble system: General set-up. Robot in stand-by position

positioned to permit the introduction of a probe towards a target, as is usually the case during stereotaxy. Any other kind of "fingers" can easily be designed according to the requirements of the task needed. A micromanipulator can be mounted to drive microelectrodes during recording sessions in functional surgery. A calibration cage made of two pairs of parallel plexiglas plates, each containing 9 lead beads, can also be mounted on the end-plate at the time of calibration, which is the initial step in all procedures.

The most important feature conferring human likeness to this robot is its "brain", which mainly houses the software used to pilot the robot. This command module is an IBM PC/AT computer, in which a designated robot programming card has been inserted. Neurosurgeons usually work in the human brain as in a cartesian space, where points are represented by the coordinates x, y, z, and a linear trajectory by two points. For the robot, the spatial coordinates of a point are a set of six different angles and even a linear trajectory between two points corresponds to a set of six complicated functions of time for its six angles. The changer matrix is a central feature of the robot's driving program. The PC is loaded with a program file which contains a calibration file, a function translating the cartesian coordinates given by the operator either through the digitizing table or the mouse of the digitized angiography system into the six angle coordinates of the robot, a file of the spatial data describing the forbidden areas (the robot's trajectory to the final target must avoid certain areas containing obstacles such as frame superstructures), and subroutine files to achieve specific purposes (such as calculations of the thalamic approach for thalamotomies or electrode implantations using ventricular landmarks: anterior and posterior commissures, top of the thalamus, midline, laterality).

2. Data Acquisition

Feeding the robot's brain with the coordinates of these targets and trajectories can be achieved through different means. i) They can be keyed as numerical values on the computer keyboard. This method can be used for small displacements of the robot, which are needed to correct, or even change, the final position of the guide-tube. ii) They can also be digitized, using a digitizing table, from X-rays obtained during the stereotactic procedure. This method is usually used when the target and the primary trajectory are defined. iii) They can also be directly taken, using a "mouse" driven cursor, from the already digitized pictures provided by a digitized substraction angiography (DSA) system. iv) Finally, they can be taken from 3 D-reconstruction[14] of a spatial target, either a space occupying lesion (such as a tumour, an abscess, a cyst, a haematoma), for biopsy or sampling or a normal structure (such as a thalamic nucleus) in the case of functional neurosurgery.

At the present time, all data are fed into the command computer via the digitizing table, from X-rays taken during the procedure. These data are of two kinds:

– calibration data: the X-ray pictures taken with the calibration cage positioned by the robot around the head of the patient show the images of the lead beads which are digitized and their coordinates introduced into the data file.

– target data: the positions of the target, or targets, which are plotted on the same pictures, are also digitized.

This system is currently being replaced by a Digitized Substracted Angiography (DSA) system (Digital Design, Saphyr system) which is used to collect all neuroradiological images, display them on monitors, and store the coordinates of every point on the images in the central DSA memory. This last feature will by-pass the steps of taking X-rays, developing films and digitizing the points of interest. Using a mouse, it is possible to move a cursor onto the target point and to sample and store the coordinates of this point. The step of the digitizing table is therefore avoided. This has the advantages of time saving, higher precision, and future possibility of automated detection of such features as the lead beads, for example.

At the present time, the complete procedure consists of the following steps: under local or general anaesthesia, depending upon the type of planned stereotaxy, the patient is placed on the frame. The four pins of the frame are inserted into burr holes through the skull and the numbers on the pin-holding verniers are recorded.

a) Calibration

The first objective of the robot is to know where it is and where the patient held by the stereotactic frame is. To achieve this, a first subroutine has been written which tells the robot to place a calibrating cage around the head of the patient. This plexiglas cage looks like an open cubic box, the four sides surrounding the aperture each being implanted with nine X-ray opaque beads, the positions of which have been precisely measured. The calibration cage is mounted on the end-plate of the robot's hand and the initial step of the program orders the robot to place the cage around the patient's head. Once the cage is placed around the head, two X-rays (frontal antero-posterior and lateral transversal) (Fig. 5) are taken which show both the lead beads and the fiducial markers of the frame on the same images. The calibration method is derived from the 2-plane method used for camera calibration[24] applied to the robot model calibration[57] using a modified Denavit-Hartenberg model[18], whose parameters were estimated using a non-linear least square algorithm. The beads appear on these films as two sets of nine dots, because of the parallax induced by the divergence of the

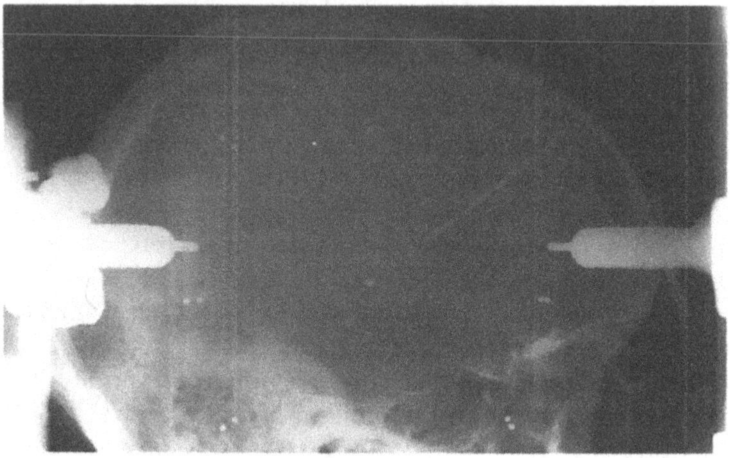

Fig. 5. The Grenoble system: the calibration cage as it appears on a lateral X-ray view: the images of the opaque beads do not superimpose due to the parallax

X-ray beams although the X-ray tubes are placed at a distance of 3.75 meters from the center of the head. When the 18 dots have been digitized, the robot software calculates both the position of the central X-ray beam and the parallax parameters. This parallax error is then automatically taken into account in all further calculations.

b) Projective Neuroradiology

This first step is followed by stereotactic projective neuroradiological examinations, including angiography and ventriculography. Angiography is performed whenever an invasive procedure is planned (biopsies, brachytherapy, cannula implantation or SEEG recording depth electrodes) except if the trajectory is systematically placed in a cortical area known (and confirmed by practice) to be avascular, such as the precoronal area used for thalamic approaches. Ventriculography is also performed in order to provide the contours and anatomical landmarks of the third ventricle on which the atlas[60, 73] references are based and which are used to calculate the thalamic targets of functional neurosurgery. Third ventricular anatomy will also be used to coordinate the stereotactic and extra-stereotactic images, such as those obtained from CT-scan and MRI pictures, which, in our set-up, are not yet possible in stereotactic conditions. In the case of a tumour, data from MRI are transfered onto the stereotactic ventriculogram and a biopsy track is chosen which is compatible with the vessels are shown on the angiograms. In the case of thalamic implantation, the target is drawn according to Guiot's diagram[70]. In all cases, the landmarks used to define the target are digitized.

c) CT-scan

The Talairach frame does not have localizers designed for MRI or CT-scan examinations in stereotactic conditions. Several solutions have been proposed to overcome this problem and to make use of the data from computerized imaging systems. When the CT-scan examination has been obtained under regular circumstances, there are several methods for extracting this information for stereotactic procedures. The simplest one, where vertical slice reconstruction is available, consists of displaying a sagittal pattern of the lesion on the scout-view. When this is enlarged to the scale of the lateral stereotactic X-ray view, superimposition of these two pictures allows the lesion profile obtained from the CT-scan to be reported in stereotactic coordinates. Nguyen *et al.*[50], have described another method when vertical slice reconstruction is not available; the head of the patient is regarded as a cube which is then sliced perpendicular to its frontal aspect. Therefore, any point on a given CT slice can be reported in the 3 D space, according to its position distance on the slice from each side of the CT picture, and to its altitude as given by the number of the slice and the space distance between two adjacent slices. Pictures can therefore be redrawn as lateral and frontal projections of the skull and of the lesion and matched to the corresponding stereotactic X-rays. We use a similar and even simpler procedure. For CT-scans, location of the slices is recognized on the basis of remarkable features (such as bony structures on the base of the skull, ventricular landmarks, calcified pineal gland, and choroid plexuses, injected vessels, etc.). This helps to position the CT-slices on the lateral X-ray. The average ratio between the distance from anterior to posterior inner tables of the skull as measured on the stereotactic lateral and frontal X-rays and that on the corresponding CT-slices is calculated and provides the magnification ratio. The distance of the antero-posterior and lateral limits of space occupying lesions is measured on the CT-slices, multiplied by the magnification ratio, and reported on the stereotactic scheme to reconstruct the pattern of the lesion[7]. The superimposition of all these different types of information constructs a final pattern on which the target and trajectory are designed and calculated. The target, along with a second point, are digitized to define the trajectory. The resident computer software computes the six angle functions necessary to drive the robot from the stand-by to final positions, taking into account all forbidden places, such as the superstructures of the frame for instance.

d) MRI

1. The problem of magnetic components of the surgical tools: Since the Talairach frame is presently built using magnetic components, magnetic resonance stereotactic imaging can not be performed with this type of frame. One must rely, therefore, on the adapters made for MRI. One can, however, reconstruct the lesion profile from the MRI images in a similar manner to that used for CT-scan. It is better to display sagittal MRI pictures enlarged at the same magnification as that of the stereotactic pictures and featuring a common landmark (cross of x-y calibration scale) allowing precisely matched superimposition of these sagittal parallel slices. The midline slice showing the third ventricle structures can be matched to the stereotactic ventriculograms. The lesion contours are then easily reported onto stereotactic maps.

2. Linearity of the MRI data: It is an often repeated statement that magnetic resonance imaging has in its basic principle the sin of non-linearity and that, as a consequence, a precise spatial localization cannot be expected from it[59, 79]. This is actually incorrect[65]. Spatial localization in MRI is a consequence of frequency coding of the space. This is achieved by applying a linear magnetic gradient which changes the main B_O field of the magnet locally and therefore changes locally the resonance frequency of the protons in a space dependant manner. The linearity of the gradients on the 3 axes X, Y, and Z may not be properly tuned and the magnification may be different along these 3 directions. This is a matter of correctly tuning the system. In the same manner, incorrect tuning of the X and Y displays on the TV screen or on the photographic reprograph can lead to a distorted final picture.

The system has to be regularly checked and eventually corrected, using a calibrated phantom. The statement that MRI measurements are inaccurate due to distorsions can apply to whole body sections where it is certain that homogeneity of the magnetic field B_O and linearity of the gradients are not correctly achieved near the walls of the gantry and also because of inhomogeneity and eddy currents. For a brain MRI examination, centered on the axis of the magnet, these distorsions can effectively be avoided. This fact needs to be stressed since MR imaging in the coming decade will be the principal source of spatial imaging of the brain and will be used for 3 D reconstruction as well as for designation of targets in the brain for computer assisted systems such as robots.

3. Transfer of data: With regard to the Talairach system, in its present commercial availability, its direct use in MRI systems is impossible. New methods of transfer of MRI data to the stereotactic space need to be designed. The easiest way is to enlarge the images at the scale of the stereotactic pictures and to match them on similarly visible features and anatomical structures.

Sedan *et al.*[62], designed a TV based system which could pick up the MRI parasagittal views and redisplay them, using a variable gain along the X and Y axis. This had the advantage of correcting the distortion of MRI images but was rather difficult to use and required special although inexpensive equipment. Recent MRI systems can actually display the pictures on the reprograph at any desired magnification. Provided that the MRI gradients are properly checked and adjusted if needed, stereotactic compatible MRI images are easily available if the neuroradiologist adds an identically positionned calibration grid to each picture. By superimposition of these grids, one may draw a composite picture featuring all relevant data, principally the inner contour of the skull, the coronal suture, the torcular depression, and the ventricular system, including the third ventricle, aqueduct of Sylvius and the 4th ventricle, as well as the rostrum and splenium of the corpus callosum, and sometimes the siphon of the carotid artery. All of these structures can also be drawn on a stereotactic diagram which can therefore be matched to the MRI scheme, and the data subsequently transfered. This procedure can be computerized.

3. General Procedure

Once the trajectory is computed, it is displayed and submitted to validation by the surgeon. Careful attention is paid to avoid any error. The difference between the recalculated and real positions of the lead beads is displayed and must be accepted by the operator before proceeding to the next step. When validation is given, the robot starts its approach. A few centimeters before reaching the final position, it stops and stands by. During this time, the robot arm and hand are dressed with a sterile plastic bag. A new validation is required and the end of the approach is made at reduced speed. If needed, the robot can be stopped instantly, at any time. X-ray controls allow verification of the current position, and if need be, correction can be made through a procedure of iterative small moves which can be triggered from the pilot computer keyboard. These moves can be performed in the cartesian space of the frame or in the six dimension angular space of the robot. Work is in progress to adjust the robot automatically to the final position via automatic detection of the image of the probe holder on digitized radiograms and comparison with the theoretical target. When the position is considered correct, the power of the command module is shut down, preventing any unexpected move of the robot during the last phase of the procedure. The robot holds its preachieved position without any possibility of change.

During the last phase, the skin is opened in front of the guide tube. A 2.3 mm hole is drilled into the skull through the guide tube and the appropriate tool (biopsy sampler, electrode, cannula, etc.) is inserted to the previously calculated depth while X-rays are taken to check the accuracy of the track (Fig. 6). For obvious security reasons during this experimental

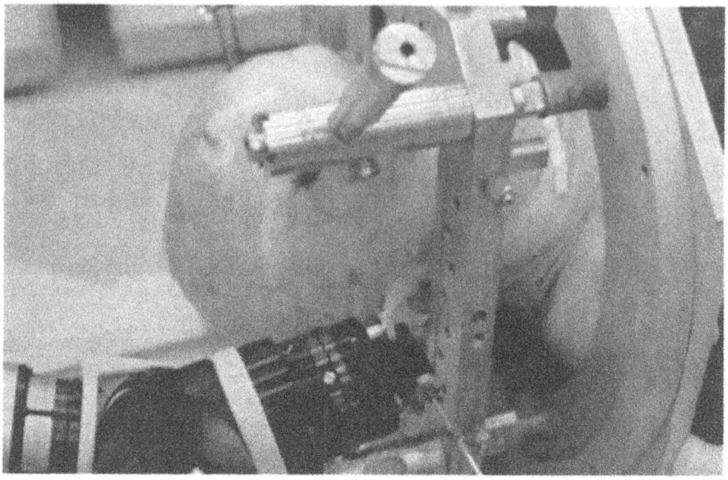

Fig. 6. The Grenoble system: The end-plate with a biopsy-probe carrier

stage of the robot's development, all penetrating procedures, although they could be performed by the robot itself, are hand made. The robot is presently used only as a guide tube holder, in order to prevent any accidents while a probe is inside the brain.

At the end of the procedure, the inserted tool is hand withdrawn and the robot is reactivated. A final subroutine drives it back to its initial resting position.

In the absence of any resistance or stress, the precision of the robot essentially depends on the zone involved by the trajectory. In most of these operation zones, the precision (defined as the precision of execution after giving spatial coordinates of the target as well as the mean deviation during repetition tests) is about a tenth of a millimeter. In some special zones, such as the left anterior temporal or at the level of the vertex, the precision is much lower and iterative displacements of about 2 or 3 mm can be required. This is due to the joint positions which have to be taken by the robot in order to achieve the required trajectory. A new program card as well as additional calibration procedures and the above mentioned automatic feedback control will reduce these inaccuracies.

No definitive statement can be made concerning limitations and drawbacks since the robot is under permanent experimental investigation and improvement. At the present time, the procedure is still rather slow due to the extensive control steps followed for obvious ethical and safety reasons. Introduction of digitized radiography will significantly shorten the duration of these steps. Dangerous steps such as drilling the skull or introduction and advancement of a tool into the brain can theoretically be

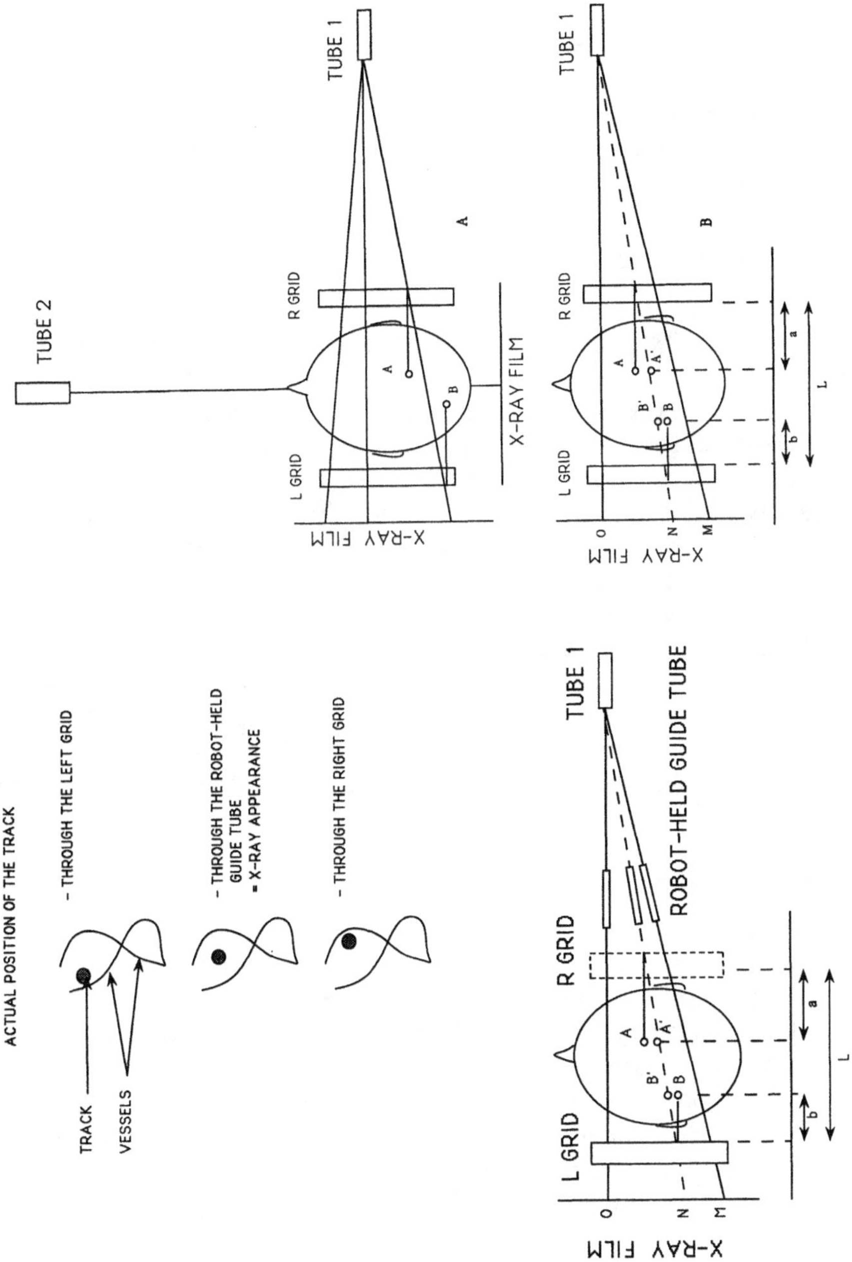

Fig. 7. Parallax errors and X-ray aligned trajectories

performed by combined six axes movements of the robot. Strain gauges are needed in order to detect changes in resistance between successive structures (bone and brain for instance) or impact against an obstacle (vessel, bone or calcified lesion). However, it is safer to use a seventh axis driven by a linear motor. Work is currently being done on this problem by the Lausanne group with possible solutions in the near future.

4. Clinical Applications

During the first 148 months of use in the stereotactic operating room, since March 1st, 1989, 208 procedures have been performed, covering the whole range of routine applications encountered in current neurosurgical practice. For the last 160 of them, the surgical team was sufficiently trained to pilot the robot without the in-room assistance of robot technicians and computer programmers. This demonstrates the level of software development, already user friendly and compatible with routine clinical use without an overly apparent experimental appearance in the operating room. The patients were informed that a robot was used, that security procedures were set up which avoided any risk, and they were told the extent and limits of its action. In all cases, they were confident and considered the robot as a new and sophisticated tool designed to improve surgery. Use of the robot did not influence patient outcomes and did not introduce any additional risk during procedures. On the contrary, the increased precision of trajectories, and the enhancement of decision due to a larger freedom of choices, often made the procedure safer.

a) Tumour Biopsies (141 cases)

Over the last several years[17, 48, 52], preliminary stereotactic investigations of brain tumours has become increasingly popular not only for diagnostic purposes using serial biopsies, but also for spatial localization before conventional neurosurgery to debulk the tumour mass or before stereotactic implantation of isotope seeds or wires for interstitial brachytherapy. In these cases, the procedure chooses a target central to the tumour core and a safest trajectory depending on the brain structures and blood vessels surrounding the tumour. In our practice, we must often use a lateral approach and choose the trajectory according to the vessels as shown in stereotactic angiography. The point representing the lateral projection of the biopsy trajectory is digitized and its coordinates are therefore available to the robot central unit in the command module which computes and proposes a trajectory which, if validated by the neurosurgeon, is executed. The guide tube is set in a position which is checked by X-rays. Once the sub-routine "Lateral approach" has calculated from he X-ray image of the calibration cage beads the position of the central X-ray beam perpendicular to the faces of the cage and along which no parallax is induced, the program can calculate the parallax error for any point not situated on this central X-ray beam. This provides the robot with the data necessary to align the guide tube along the X-ray beam passing by the target point, with the advantage of creating a trajectory colinear to this X-ray beam which will have the same relationships with the surrounding structures, such as blood vessels, shown on the X-ray picture (Fig. 7). If needed, iterative displacements of the guide tube can be achieved via the keyboard of the driving computer which allows one to chose from a menu the amplitude (from 0 to 100 mm with a 0.1 mm precision) of the displacements, the x, y and z axis on which they are desired, and their speed (from 5% to 100% of the maximal speed).

In 116 patients, this lateral approach has been used to take 350 samples. In 25 patients, a double oblique trajectory (as described below) was used, mainly to reach tumours of the midline such as in the pineal region or in the third ventricle. In these cases, it is easy to choose the best trajectory, for example passing through a foramen of Monro and ending at the center of the cyst or tumour. Positioning of a ventriculoscope would also be significantly easier with the robot, particularly when several tracks are needed.

b) Stereo-electro-encephalographic (SEEG) Investigations of Epileptic Patients (14 cases)

Stereo-electro-encephalography (SEEG) consists of introducing into the brain of an epileptic patient several depth electrodes with 5 to 15 contacts in a row, at precise locations depending on the clinical features of the epileptic seizures and aimed at determining the extent of the epileptic focus and of its propagating paths, with a view to surgical excision[2, 11, 51, 72]. These sites are chosen according to these clinical considerations as well as to the permitted areas based on the angiograms. They are digitized in the same way as for lateral biopsies and the guide tube is positioned by the robot as previously described. The robot has a special subroutine which provides the possibility to feed the program with all the desired sites of SEEG electrode implantation (usually 5 to 10, with sometimes 1 contralateral electrode) at the same time and of subsequently positioning the guide tube. As for biopsies, drilling the holes, insertion of holding screws through the guide, and insertion of the electrodes into the central hole of the screws are still performed manually. 14 patients underwent this procedure and had 107 electrodes inserted in this way.

c) Brachytherapy (5 cases)

Introduction of permanent ^{125}I seeds or ^{192}Ir wires is very similar, in terms of stereotactic procedure, to biopsy sampling and has been performed 5 times in this series of robot-operated patients. ^{125}I brachytherapy (3 patients) in our protocol is performed by permanent implantation of a single seed of 12.5 mCi of ^{125}I to deliver 60 Gys over a 35 mm diameter spherical surface in small low grade gliomas. Brachytherapy with ^{192}Ir is very similar to SEEG investigations as it requires the insertion of removable adjustable catheters[4, 25, 67] and has been performed in 2 patients of this series (1 by lateral approach and 1 by oblique approach). The possibility to position the robot guide tube at any desired distance from the scalp makes this procedure, as well as SEEG electrode insertion, much easier than using the conventional grids of the Talairach frame which require the design of specific devices[11, 51].

d) Midline Stereotactic Neurosurgery

Oblique approaches are needed mainly when the target is in the midline area, either for biopsies of midline tumours (pineal gland, third ventricle area), or for functional surgery of the basal ganglia (Parkinson's disease, chronic pain).

We used this approach to treat 2 patients with deafferentation pain by chronic somatosensory thalamic stimulation and 34 patients suffering from dyskinesias (29 Parkinson's disease and 5 dyskinesias of other origins) by permanent thalamic VIM (ventral intermedius nucleus) stimulation. As the disease is often bilateral, 46 thalamic sites were implanted in this series of patients. The interest in using a robot is particularly well demonstrated in this type of procedure. The target, mainly the VIM nucleus in our dyskinesia patients[5, 6, 70, 75], is principally defined on the basis of anatomical landmarks (the anterior and posterior commissures of the third ventricle, the top of the thalamus and the midline) using a geometrical paradigm[70] and given lateralities[75]. A subroutine has been written which computes the VIM spatial coordinates from these landmarks as digitized on the ventriculograms and then positions the robot. Control X-rays are taken with a mock-probe inserted into the guide tube against the skin and corrective displacements can be performed if needed. This saves a considerable amount of time, especially when bilateral electrodes are inserted. During the procedure, the exact target is precisely located using a first trajectory, based on the same landmarks, which crosses the VIM nucleus while recognizing its boundaries by semi-microelectrode recording. A further step in robotization of this procedure is in progress which will drive the electrode micromanipulator from the robot computer and will report the calculated position of the electrode tip on the ventriculogram as well as on stereotactic atlas maps.

e) Operative Complications

Only complications relevant to the use of the robot in the above described procedures are mentionned here. Surgical complications due to biopsy sampling, electrode introduction, isotope implantation or deep brain stimulation, when they happen, as well as the therapeutic results of these procedures, cannot be attributed to the use of the robot. In this series of 113 patients, we did not observe any complication which would have been eventually induced by the use of a robot. Positioning was always possible as intended with the expected precision, in the limits of visual detectability in X-ray controls by the surgeon's eye. There was no displacement of the guide tube during penetrating procedures (nor any unwanted displacement during previous steps when the robot was not deactivated). In addition, there was no limitation in the execution of the intended program due to robot use itself.

It is important to note that during this clinical experience the robot was found to be as safe as conventional stereotactic procedures. Moreover, the flexibility of its positioning made the choice of trajectories easier and thus, the overall procedure safer.

5. Perspectives

This chapter describes the state of the art of robotics in our neurosurgical department as currently performed in the daily routine. Future perspectives which have recently been presented in the literature on robotics in medicine are applicable, and for some of them adaptation to our system is in progress. In general terms, future perspectives of neurosurgical robotics include solutions to the current problems of neurosurgery and stereotaxy, such as automatic adjustment of positioning, comparison with data-bases (including atlases), use of 3 D images, detection of the possible presence of vessels in a chosen trajectory. The links, inherent to robots, with powerful computers make these solutions now available.

a) Short Term Perspectives

1. Seventh axis: Penetration of the probe could be driven by the robot even in the present state of development. However, the robot's linear advance has not been refined to within millimetric precision, because the method used to generate linear advance involves iterative computation of a succession of points on a line. New software will allow the generation of a more linear trajectory, which could be used to drive a probe into the brain. However, another solution is more easily available. On the "wrist" of the robot, the sterilizable tool, which is at the present time a guide tube, can be replaced by a motorized tool, such as a drill or a micromanipulator used for the insertion of a biopsy sampler, an electrode, or a cannula. The final positioning of the probe can therefore be driven by the computer and integrated into the general software of the robot. This will be particularly interesting by providing feedback input on the spatial localization data of the tip of the probe and its display on X-rays, operating diagrams, or stereotactic brain atlas maps.

2. Digitization and automated adjustment: Digitized X-ray images have already been used in stereotaxy[54]. At the present time, the data are taken from X-rays (angiograms, ventriculograms) by manual digitization of landmarks on a digitizing table. A Digital Design image processor (Saphyr) has been set up in the operating room and processes the images taken by a fluoroscope (28 cms in diameter) and a Hamamatsu TV camera. The data provided on X-ray films and manually digitized are now directly available from the digital data bank of the image processor and can be sampled on the video display using a mouse driven cursor. An automated procedure is being set up to recognize the images of the calibration cage lead beads and perform the calibration step automatically. A similar approach is possible for detecting the image of the hole of the guide tube, comparing it with the designated position, and computing the necessary iterative displacements in order to adjust the final position of the guide tube exactly as desired.

3. Computer-resident atlas: This was among the first applications of computers to neurosurgery[30]. The basal ganglia area of the Schaltenbrand atlas[60] has been digitized and the various anatomical structures have been named. An algorithm involving 3 D-spline functions has been designed[14] and provides 3 D reconstruction of these structures. The planned or actual trajectories can be displayed on these maps as intersections of the track with every plate or as a recalculated plane including the whole track.

b) Middle Term Perspectives

1. Use of 3 D images: 3 D reconstruction algorithms[14] have been successfully applied to MRI and CAT-scan images. Connection of the Image Processor of the operating room with the VAX computer of the Department of Computer Sciences will make possible the matching of these 3 D images with the stereotactic X-ray images in the operating room. The direct choice of the target from MRI and CAT-scan pictures of the pathological target will therefore be possible.

2. Detection of vascular impacts along a double oblique biopsy track: A further step is planned to recognize the blood vessels and detect the theoretical hit points between them and the intended trajectory. This will provide an aid to decision making. Current approaches to solve this important problem are detailed[7] elsewhere[13, 15, 63, 66, 77].

Vascular impact on a biopsy track must have the same Z altitudes on frontal and lateral X-rays. However, intersection points between vessels and the track on frontal and lateral views may suggest a false impact. Although this test leads to excess detection of such impacts, it is safe and must be complemented by an expert surgeon's analysis in order to distinguish false and true potential impacts. Any penetrating trajectory into the brain presents a high risk of vascular impact which is particularly important in the case of biopsies. Biopsy tracks which are aligned along the X-ray axes, i.e. either lateral or frontal approaches, provide the safest procedures, since it it possible to check on the corresponding X-ray images that the projected track which appears as a point does not correspond to any projection of a vessel. This is the most frequent circumstance in the Talairach system which is mainly set up for these orthogonal, frontal, or lateral approaches. In the case of double oblique approaches, the problem of vascular impact detection is not easy to solve. Despite the fact that CT-guided stereotactic biopsies without angiographic control are becoming increasingly popular, the theoretical risk of hitting and damaging a vessel with the biopsy cannula persists as is demonstrated by occasional bleeding complications. Effective solutions have to be found and some of them have already been designed and used. The intrinsic features of the Talairach system have led Szikla *et al.*[68, 69], to design a routine procedure, proven to be efficient and quite simple to perform, which requires no computation but can easily be computerized and automated. Provided that the two X-ray beams are orthogonal, a given point in the brain appears on X-rays as two couples of coordinates (x, z) on the frontal view and (y, z) on the lateral view, z being the same in both couples. Therefore, the projections of the intersection of a putative track with a vessel must have the same z value (as measured on X-ray films from the base plate of the frame) on both lateral and frontal planes. Obviously, the reciprocal is not true and it may happen that lateral and frontal intersections having a same z do not correspond to the same vessel. In this case, the decision between true and false potential impact is made by the surgeon's expertise which has proven to be satisfactory and is used daily in the routine practice of stereotacticians. This analysis can easily be computerized on digitized angiograms on which the theoretical track is projected by the computer which can calculate the coincidence on both projections of the intersections between the track and the vessels and display as hyper-brilliant points the intersections with similar z. These hyper-brilliant points will comprise not only the true but also those which are false potential impacts which, in a first phase, can be deleted by the surgeon's expertise.

A second method[46] is to compute and display on the two orthogonal views the theoretical trajectory and two extreme points K and L which will appear as (K′, L′) and (K″, L″) (Fig. 8). The intersection points between the vessels and the projected lines can be fully described using an index ranging from 0 to 1, 0 corresponding to K and 1 to L for instance. Every

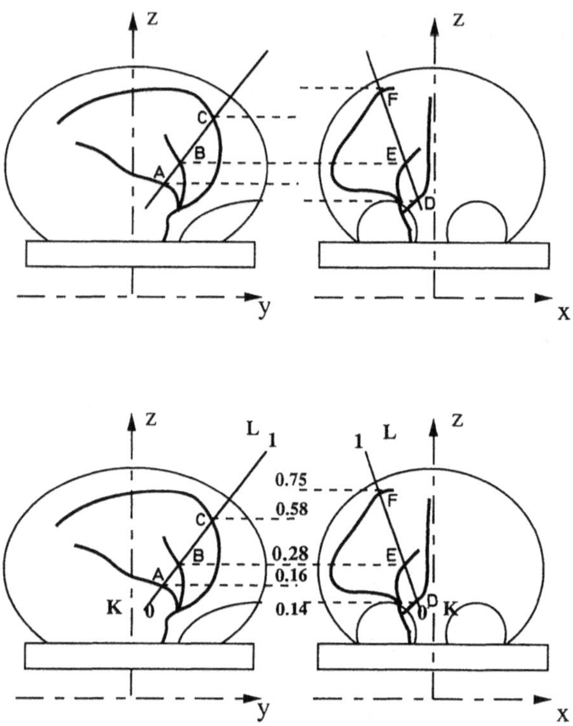

Fig. 8. Oblique tracks and vascular impacts

true impact must have similar lateral and frontal index values. Obviously false impacts will be detected by this paradigm and will be deleted by the surgeon's "expert system" analysis as easily and efficiently as in the previous case. This is evidently less elegant than true impact detection without false positive points which can be expected from real 3 D reconstruction of the vascular network, but is also much easier and faster to perform.

– 3 D evaluation of vessel position by stereoscopic analysis (double incidence angiography):

A first approach is provided by the "floating line" concept[15]. A specially built stereocomparator features two movable lines on transparent grids, applied on the two stereoscopic angiograms and representing the projection on these tilted angiograms of a theoretical line in the brain space. Observation of this line through the stereocomparator allows the surgeon to check eventual impact of the line with vessels and eventually to change it.

The Talairach system provides another approach which has been used to advantage in routine practice[67] to recognize the in depth position of the vessels using small angle-double incidence angiograms (SADIA) taken under a 5 ° tilt angle, corresponding to the natural binocular angle. One may use a stereocomparator or, with some training, it is possible to squint and obtain a 3 D perception of the vascular network. One may also superimpose the two angiograms and try to make the vessels correspond. From experience, it appears that coincidence of the two images of the vessels is only possible for those which are in the same plane perpendicular to the X-ray axis. Slightly sliding the films one over the other will change this "coincidence plane" and display another array of vessels situated within it. This is easily used in daily routine to evaluate the depth of vessels projecting on an proposed trajectory. This can also be more formally computed as follows.

– attempt to design a paradigm for computerized 3 D vascular reconstruction:

Obviously, the above described approach can be formally demonstrated and could be used as a possible basis for 3 D reconstruction. If we consider lateral views taken as SADIAs, every point P of the brain is assigned a triplet of coordinates (x, y, z) in the brain space, a pair of coordinates (Y, Z) on the regular lateral view film, and (Y′, Z′) on the lateral view film of the 5° tilted head. Therefore, x corresponds to the "depth" of a point along an axis Ox perpendicular to the film plane. When the two films are superimposed with a given shift δ, with respect to an arbitrary reference ($Y + \delta = Y'$), two sets of points belonging to the two films are placed in coincidence. Is there any relationship between δ and x? Is this relationship independent of y?

i) Coordinates of a point P in the referential of the X-ray system:

Any point P in the brain space can be described using either cartesian coordinates x, y, z or spherical coordinates ρ, α, θ where ρ is the modulus of the vector OP, α the angle between OP and the horizontal plane xOy, and θ the angle between OP and the vertical plane yOz.

$$\begin{aligned} x &= \rho \cdot \cos\alpha \cdot \sin\theta \\ y &= \rho \cdot \cos\alpha \cdot \cos\theta \\ z &= \rho \cdot \sin\alpha \end{aligned}$$

If the frame is rotated along the body axis of the patient by an angle $\Delta\theta$ such as:

$$\theta' = \theta + \Delta\theta$$

then, the point P has in the X-ray referential the new coordinates x′, y′, z′:

$$\begin{aligned} x' &= \rho \cdot \cos\alpha \cdot \sin\theta' \\ y' &= \rho \cdot \cos\alpha \cdot \cos\theta' \\ z' &= \rho \cdot \sin\alpha = z \end{aligned}$$

This can be expressed by a rotation matrix:

$$\begin{pmatrix} x' \\ y' \\ z' \end{pmatrix} = \begin{pmatrix} \cos\Delta\theta & -\sin\Delta\theta & 0 \\ \sin\Delta\theta & \cos\Delta\theta & 0 \\ 0 & 0 & 1 \end{pmatrix} \cdot \begin{pmatrix} x \\ y \\ z \end{pmatrix}$$

ii) Coordinates of projections of the point P on the X-ray film:

Due to the divergence of the X-ray beams, D being the distance from the X-ray tube to the center of the head and d the distance from this center to the X-ray film, the magnification coefficient G(x) of the X-ray pictures is:

$$G(x) = \frac{D + d}{D + x}$$

G(x) depends on the value of x, which changes when the head is tilted. Then:

$$Y = y \cdot \frac{D + d}{D + x}$$

There is a similar relationship between Z and z, even when x is changed into x′, then:

$$\begin{pmatrix} Y \\ Z \end{pmatrix} = \begin{pmatrix} \dfrac{D + d}{D + x} \end{pmatrix} \cdot \begin{pmatrix} y \\ z \end{pmatrix}$$

and

$$\begin{pmatrix} Y' \\ Z' \end{pmatrix} = \begin{pmatrix} \dfrac{D + d}{D + x'} \end{pmatrix} \cdot \begin{pmatrix} y' \\ z' \end{pmatrix}$$

iii) Relationship between x and δ:

When the films are superimposed, some structures, such as vessels can be matched on both films when there is a shift between the two films equal to δ:

**) Simple case of no magnification, with parallel x-rays: G(x) = 1 or dG(x)/dx = 0. Then:

$$\begin{aligned} \delta &= y - y' \\ &= \rho \cdot \cos\alpha \cdot [\cos\theta' - \cos\theta] \\ &= -2\sin\frac{\Delta\theta}{2}\left[x \cdot \cos\frac{\Delta\theta}{2} + y \cdot \sin\frac{\Delta\theta}{2}\right] \end{aligned}$$

$$\Delta\theta = 5°$$

Let's call:

$$b = \cos\frac{\Delta\theta}{2} = 0.999048$$

and

$$a = \sin\frac{\Delta\theta}{2} = 0.0436$$

Then:

$$x = -\frac{1}{2ab}\cdot[\delta + y\cdot a^2]$$

and, in our set-up:

$$x = -12.5\,\delta - 0.02\,y$$

**) Regular case with non parallel x-rays, where magnification G(x) depends on x, i.e. $dG(x)/dx \neq 0$. Then:

One may show that (7):

$$x = -11.9\,\delta - 0.04\,y$$

The depth x can therefore be calculated, for all points of the film which are situated at the coordinate Y and coincident to their homologous projection on the tilted film when the shift is equal to δ. A paradigm can be derived from this procedure, in several steps:

1) Digitization of the regular angiogram, attributing a set of coordinates (Y_i, Z_i) to the points Pi of the vascular network projection.

2) Digitization of the tilted angiogram, attributing a new set of coordinates (Y_i', Z'_i) to the points Pi of the vascular network projection.

3) Application to the set of coordinates (Y_i, Z_i) a shift δ along the Y axis and detection of the points Pi verifying the relationship:

$(Y_i + \delta, Z_i) = (Y_i', Z'_i)$.

For these points, according to the previously demonstrated equations, once the corresponding values of x_i, and therefore of:

$$G(x) = \frac{D + d}{D + x}$$

are calculated, y_i and z_i may be calculated from Y_i and Z_i.

A complete set of coordinates (x_i, y_i, z_i) is therefore generated and, when displayed, provides a 3 D reconstruction of the vascular network.

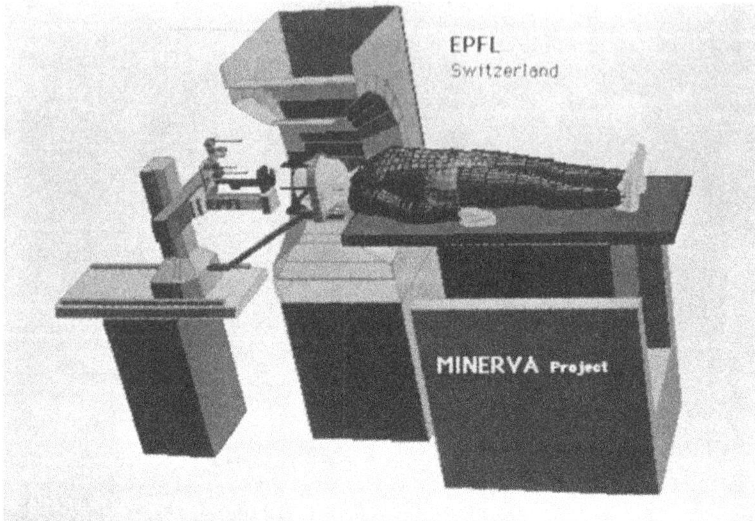

Fig. 9. The Lausanne system: computer simulation of the stereotactic robot in the gantry of the CT-scanner. (With permission of the authors)

A.3. The Lausanne System (Fig. 9)

This system[22] is mainly dedicated to the development of peripheral tools. Initially designed as a robot aimed at working in the gantry of a CAT-scanner, it can be considered also as a complement of an anthropomorphic robot which handles the surgical probes (drill, cannulae, electrodes, etc). To achieve its goals, its specifications include the following features:

– The whole stereotactic procedure is performed inside the CAT-scanner gantry.

– Subsequent CAT-scans can be performed during surgery without interference with the procedure.

– It is compatible with a non-dedicated CAT-scanner.

– The complete procedure, including skin incision, burrhole drilling and instrument changes, is made by the robot.

Prototypes of all the parts have been designed and are presently being tested in the laboratory. The stereotactic frame and the robot base are linked together in a completely rigid manner and move together with the CAT-table. This set-up is similar to that of the Kwoh-Young system. The robot has five units which include the arm, the wrist, the skin penetrating unit, the probe positioner, and the probe stocking unit. All probes have the same connecting system to fit the probe stocking unit. The combined functions of all units allow orientation along the stereotactic trajectory, as well as axial movements to penetrate the skin, drill the bone, and insert the probes. Safety is provided by manual reversibility in case of power failure. During the procedure, a cutting guide tube is initially advanced down to the bone. Through this are subsequently introduced a skin evacuator, a drill, a dura perforator, and then straight and side-outlet electrodes. A personal computer takes over the non-compressed data from the CAT-scanner. Target selection is performed on a larger computer housing a resident atlas, which generates and transmits the commands to the robot control unit.

B. Stereotactically Guided Open-field Surgical Robots

Two systems use robotized microscopes to position the optical axis, and the surgical approach to the lesion and even participate in the treatment phase.

B.1. The Mayo Clinic System (Fig.10)

This system is undoubtedly the first example of routine clinical application of an integrated computerized system bringing together CT and MRI imaging, target computation from 3 D reconstruction of the tumour, robotized command of a surgical tool (in the present case, a laser beam guided through a microscope), and image guided removal of the lesion. To over-

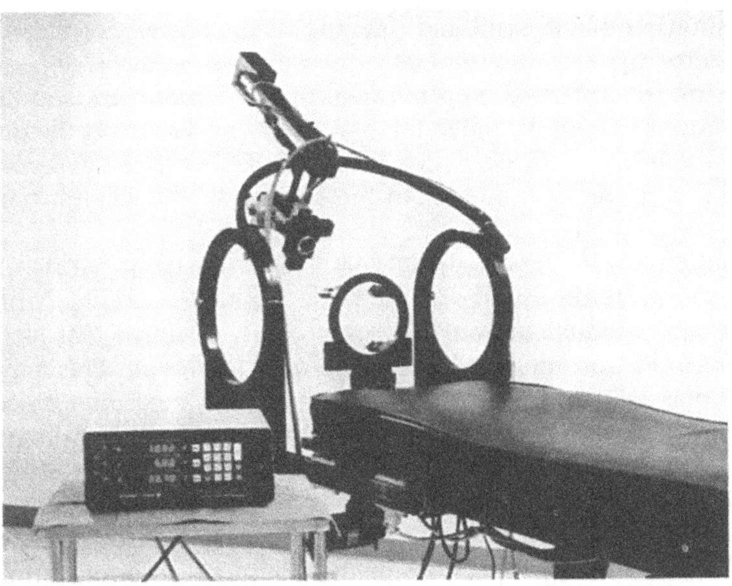

Fig. 10. The Mayo Clinic system: general set-up. (With permission of the authors)

come the neurosurgical inability to recognize the limits of tumours precisely as well as to maintain surgical orientation within an irregularly shaped and deep seated lesion, the authors of this system designed and used a stereotactically directed and computer monitored carbon dioxide laser for precision resection of CT-defined tumours located in 3D space by CT-scan and MRI performed in stereotactic conditions.

Within a 3D computer matrix, a 3D data base is constructed from stereotactically acquired CT and MRI images of the tumour limits. The data tapes are read into a Data General Eclipse S 140 computer system located in the operating room where CT and MRI images are displayed on a Ramster raster scan terminal. An automatic intensity detection program as well as the use of the system cursor allows one to digitize the localization reference marks and multiple points along the margins of the tumour on each CT and MRI slice. A solid volume in stereotactic space is created and displayed using a shaded graphics program as a tumour volume or slice orthogonal to any surgical approach. The computer also places the center of the tumour at the focal point of the arc quadrant stereotactic frame by means of a motorized X, Y, Z slide. An operating microscope and laser micromanipulator box (optically coupled to a Sharplan 743 CO2 surgical laser) are attached to a carriage mounted on an double gimbled arc attached to the base of the frame. A digital readout system displays the distance of the microscope and laser focal points from the focal point of the stereotactic frame, measured by optical encoders and slices cut orthogonal to the surgical approach at the level of microscope/laser focal points are also displayed on the terminal.

Trephination of the skull and opening of the cortex are therefore precisely directed towards the tumour core and possible displacements of the brain during the approach and removal of the tumour are checked using teleradiograms of metallic balls stereotactically placed along the track. The tumour is vaporized slice by slice using 65–85 Watts of defocused laser power in a continuous mode, from the surface to the deepest part of the tumour.

226 patients were reported in 1988[33] suffering from various types of brain tumours. In about 70% of the patients, post-operative controls did not show any residual tumour. In some cases, a subsequent stereotactic laser procedure accomplished apparent total removal. The majority of glioblastomas who underwent total removal had local recurrence within 3–11 months following surgery. Although this confirms that the prognosis of glioblastomas is not related to the extent of the surgical excision, the tremendous interest of the Mayo Clinic approach resides in the possibility of planning of total and image guided resection of a deep seated lesion. This had a determining impact on the development of robotic applications to neurosurgery[41].

B.2. The Grenoble-Paris-Rennes Robotized Microscope (Fig. 11)

Using a similar approach to that of Kelly, we designed a robot-held microscope which is based on a triple arm parallel system, attached to the ceiling of the operating room and which is able to hold the operating microscope in a given position, to move this microscope either by finite displacements driven from a joystick, a pedal-set, or a keyboard, or to follow the operator's intention through strain-gauge equipped handles which are held by the surgeon. In this mode, the servomechanisms driving the microscope make a strain-speed conversion and the apparent weight and stiffness of the system are minimized. Since the encoders of the different joints of the robot know at every moment the exact position of the robot, this system is perfectly suited to be coupled to an image data base which would allow command of the position of the microscope from the brain 3 D images and from lesion localization. At this stage, the system would resemble the Kelly system and would allow open field computer assisted neurosurgery. At the present time, the system is only servo-assisted for "zero-gravity like" handling.

C. Positioning Robots

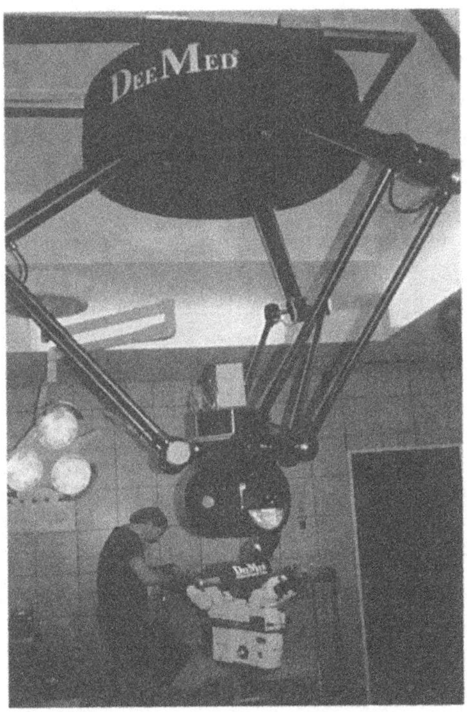

Fig. 11. The G.P.R robot microscope holder

C.1. The "Neuronavigator"

An articulated neurosurgical navigation system using MRI and CT images has been designed and is now commercially available[42]. It is a six angle passively activated arm, attached to the Mayfield head holder and the finger tip of which can be passively positioned by the operator into a given site in the brain. The system has been previously calibrated by pin-pointing three anatomical features of the patient such as the nasion, and tragus. The computer is fed with the image data base corresponding to the operated patient. The software is able to recalculate the position of the finger tip and to display it on the CT or MR slices, enabling the neurosurgeon to know at any moment where he is in the brain space of his patient. This concept has already been used by Patrick Kelly who reports in his microscope visual field the recalculated theoretical image of the lesion at the level the surgeon is supposed to be operating on at any given moment. Such a system as the neuronavigator could obviously be of great help during surgical procedures in allowing the surgeon to control the extent and situation of his acts.

C.2. The Retractor Robot

In a similar manner, a retractor held by a robot has been recently designed by the Toronto group, aimed at positioning and controlling the applied pressure against the brain parenchyma.

III.2. Robots in Other Medical Fields

A. Ophthalmology

A micro-manipulator like system is designed to perform delicate procedures on the eye-ball[78]. Micro-tools have also been designed but there is presently no feed-back to an image data bank which would allow the system to act intelligently with respect to knowledge of the spatial shape, size, or situation of a lesion or anatomical structure.

B. Robot Assisted Nursing Care

Although these systems belong more to the "domotic" domain than to the field of computer assisted neurosurgery, it is evident that robot machines capable of transfering patients from their bed to the operating table or to examination table, such as neuroradiology tables for instance, as well as helping rehabilitation teams or even compensating patients deficits, would be very useful. A study of the market and possible applications is currently being adressed in the literature and in scientific meetings (Biostim 90, Nice, June 1990).

IV. Future Applications and Science-fiction

IV.1. Open Surgery

The final goal of computer assisted surgery is to achieve intraoperative control of surgical tool position with respect to the pathological lesion, such as tumour. As a result of stereotactic investigations, the tumour is precisely located with respect to the fiducial markers of the frame. It is therefore possible to place the patient in an operating frame and take advantage of a surgical robot for the tasks of spatial localization and guiding the surgeon's tools during "open field" surgery. This is in the same perspective as Kelly's approach[35, 36] which has already demonstrated the advantages of such a procedure[28, 31, 32, 37, 41]. Intermediate solutions have also been reported to guide surgical trephination[42, 56] or during the intracerebral procedure, using ultrasound localization[10, 27, 47, 76].

IV.2. Flexible Robots

The achievement of flexible robots capable of moving a snake-shaped body between a network of obstacles, keeping in memory the position of these obstacles is perfectly adapted to the goal of moving a clip into an anatomically complex environment, such as the surroundings of an aneurysm of the middle cerebral artery. This will allow deep and ill placed targets to be reached but also will call for the parallel development of vision systems to monitor what happens at the tip of the flexible robot which will usually be hidden from the direct sight of the neurosurgeon.

IV.3. Sensor Guided Robots

In addition to vision, which is needed to provide the neurosurgeon with the possibility to control the act being done, it can be imagined that the robot would need additional information to achieve its task. It would need to be fed with data about pressure, tissue resistance and stiffness, ultrasound reflectivity, electrical impedance, and so on. This also implies that the robot would be equipped with expert systems capable of processing these data and making decisions from them. Although this is probably not possible to day, we cannot assume that it will be still impossible tomorrow.

V. Discussion and Conclusion

The stereotactic robot should be considered as a first step in the more general approach of computer assisted medico-surgical procedures. The development of such a system opens the way to an integrated system linking image databases, theoretical reference databases (such as computer-resident stereotactic atlases), and surgical procedures, during either stereotactic or "open surgery". The long term goal is to build an interactive system allowing surgical procedures during which the surgeon knows at every moment where he is, what he is doing, and what structures his acts involve via a feedback mechanism in which the data banks are continually fed with new information gathered during the procedure.

The future of robotics in neurosurgery needs to be considered carefully. As the forthcoming development of this methodology accelerates and as industry becomes more and more interested in robot technology, the size of the market will stimulate progress in this field which in turn will open the way for new applications which cannot be performed at the present time due to technological limitations. All medical technologies have benefited from this kind of process. Recent improvements in endoscopic methods have permitted new neurosurgical applications, but are presently limited by the inaccessibility of deep structures. The increased dexterity provided by robotization will make possible what today is considered utopia. Related fields such as engineering, optics, biomaterials, artificial vision, and miniaturization will contribute to the conception and realization of flexible robots, holding sensors (ultra-sonic, barometric or visual) capable of driving themselves along winding trajectories amidst deep and fragile anatomical landscapes, such as the Sylvian fissures, the basal cisterns and the ventricular cavities, towards deep seated, small sized or even moving targets.

At every step of this evolution, the double imperatives of decreasing invasiveness and increasing precision and efficiency must be kept in mind. Although robot technology will push back the frontiers of the feasable, the time has not yet come for imposing the three laws of robotics stated by Isaac Asimov[1], which make a robot unable to harm a human being, obliged to obey human orders when they do not jeopardize the first law, and committed to protect itself as long as the first two laws are respected. Neither can a robot be heard asking why the surgeon bothered coming into the operating room. Despite the wildest neurosurgery-fiction fantasies, robots will be here for nothing more than helping and serving the surgeon.

References

1. Asimov I (1950) I, Robot. Doubleday, New York
2. Bancaud J, Talairach J, Bonis A, Schaub C, Szikla G, Morel P, Bordas-Ferrer H (1965) La stéreo-électro-encéphalographie dans l'épilepsie. Masson, Paris
3. Benabid AL, Cinquin P, Lavallée S, Le Bas JF, Demongeot J, de Rougemont J (1987) Computer-driven robot for stereotactic surgery connected to CT scan and magnetic resonance imaging. Appl Neurophysiol 50: 153–154
4. Benabid AL, Chirossel JP, Mercier C, Louveau A, Passagia JG, Henry S, de Rougemont J, Vrousos C (1987) Removable, adjustable and reusable implants for stereotactic interstitial radiosurgery of brain tumours. Appl Neurophysiol 50: 278–280

5. Benabid AL, Pollak P, Louveau A, Henry S, de Rougemont J (1987) Combined (thalamotomy and stimulation) stereotactic surgery of the VIM thalamus nucleus for bilateral Parkinson disease. Appl Neurophysiol 50: 344–346
6. Benabid AL, Pollak P, Hommel M, Gaio JM, de Rougemont J, Perret J (1989) Traitement du tremblement parkinsonien par stimulation chronique du noyau ventral intermediaire du Thalamus. Rev Neurol (Paris) 145: 320–323
7. Benabid AL, Lavallée S, Hoffmann D, Cinquin P, Le Bas JF, Demongeot J (1991) The Talairach system. In: Kelly PJ (ed) Computers in stereotactic neurosurgery. Blackwell Scientific Publication, Cambridge (in press)
8. Benabid AL, Lavallée S, Hoffmann D, Cinquin P, Demongeot J, Danel F (1991) Computer driven robot for stereotactic neurosurgery. In: Kelly PJ (ed) Computers in stereotactic neurosurgery. Blackwell Scientific Publication, Cambridge (in press)
9. Benabid AL, Lavallée S, Hoffmann D, Cinquin P, Demongeot J, Danel F (1991) Potential use of robots in endoscopic neurosurgery. Acta Neurochir (Wien) (in press)
10. Berger MS (1986) Ultrasound-guided stereotaxic biopsy using a new apparatus. J Neurosurg 65: 550–554
11. Bouvier G, Saint Hilaire JM, Giard N, Lesage J, Cloutier L, Beique R (1987) Depth electrode implantation at Hospital Notre-Dame, Montreal. In: Engel J Jr (ed) Surgical treatment of the epilepsies. Raven Press, New York, pp 589–594
12. Brown RA (1979) A computerized tomography-computer graphics approach to stereotactic localization. J Neurosurg 50: 715–720
13. Camillerapp J, Leplumey J, Walter A (1987) Acquisition of a 3 D model of the cranial vascular system from two stereoscopic pictures. AFCET; 16–20 Nov, 1987; Antibes
14. Cinquin P (1987) Application des fonctions splines au traitement d'images numériques. Thèse d'ètat de Sciences Mathématiques; Université Joseph Fourier, Grenoble
15. Cloutier L, Nguyen DN, Ghosh S, Boulianne M, Labissonniére P, Bouvier G, Beique R (1985) Simulator allowing spatial viewing of cerebral probes by using a floating line concept. Symposium on optical and electro-optical applied science and Engineering. Cannes, France
16. Colombo F, Angrilli F, Zanardo A, Pinna V, Alexandre A, Benedetti A (1982) A universal method to employ CT scanner spatial information in stereotactic surgery. Appl Neurophysiol 45: 352–354
17. Daumas-Duport C, Monsaingeon V, Szenthe L, Szikla G (1982) Serial stereotactic biopsies: a double histological code of gliomas according to malignancy and 3 D configuration, as an aid to therapeutic decision and assessment of results. Appl Neurophysiol 45: 431–437
18. Denavit J, Hartenberg RS, Evanston ILL (1955) A kinematic notation for lower-pair mechanisms based on matrices. J Appl Mech 55: 215–221
19. Doll J, Schlegel W, Pastyr O, Sturm V, Maier-Borst W (1987) The use of an industrial robot as a stereotactic guidance system. CAR' 79: 374–378
20. Gildenberg PL (1987) Whatever happened to stereotactic surgery? Neurosurg 20: 983–987

21. Gildenberg PL. Kaufmann HH, Krishna Murthy KS (1982) Calculation of stereotactic coordinates from the computed tomographic scan. Appl Neurophysiol 45: 443–448
22. Glauser D, Flury P, Durr P, Funakubo H, Burckhardt CW, Favre J, Schnyder P, Fankhauser H (1990) Configuration of a robot dedicated to stereotactic surgery. Stereotactic and Functional Neurosurgery 54 + 55: 468–470
23. Goerss SJ, Kelly PJ, Kall BA, Alker GJ (1982) A computed tomographic stereotactic adaptation system. Neurosurgery 10: 375–379
24. Gremban KD, Thorpe CE, Kanade T (1988) Geometric camera calibration using systems of linear equations. Proc IEEE of Int Conf on Robotics and Automation, Philadelphia, pp 947–951
25. Gutin PH, Phillips TL, Wara WM, Leibel SA, Hosobuchi Y, Leven VA, Weaver KA, Lamb S (1984) Brachytherapy of recurrent malignant brain tumours with removable high activity iodine-125 sources. J Neurosurg 60: 61–68
26. Horsley VA, Clarke RH (1905) On the intrinsic fibers of the cerebellum, its nuclei and its effect tracts. Brain 28: 12–29
27. Iseki H, Amano K (1985) CT-guided stereotactic surgery in combination with intra-operative monitoring by sector type ultrasonography. Asian Med J 28: 157–167
28. Kall BA, Kelly PJ, Goerss SJ (1985) Interactive stereotactic surgery system for the removal of intracranial tumours utilizing the CO2 laser and the CT-derived database. IEEE Trans Biomed Eng 32: 112–116
29. Kall BA, Kelly PJ, Goerss SJ, Earnest F (1985) IV. Cross-registration of points and lesions volumes from MR and CT. Proceed. 7° annual meeting of frontiers of engineering and computing in health care, pp 935–942
30. Kall BA, Kelly PJ, Goerss SJ, Frieder G (1985) Methodology and clinical experience with computed tomography and a computer-resident stereotactic atlas. Neurosurgery 17: 400–407
31. Kall BA, Kelly PJ, Goerss S (1987) Comprehensive computer assisted data collection treatment planning and interactive surgery. Proceed. SPIE, Medical imaging 767: 509–514
32. Kelly PJ (1986) Technical approaches to identification and stereotactic reduction of tumour burden. In: Walker MD, Thomas DGT (eds) Biology of brain tumour. Martinus Nijhoff, Boston Dordrecht Lancaster, pp 237–343
33. Kelly PJ (1988) Volumetric stereotactic surgical resection of intraaxial brain mass lesions. Mayo Clinic Proc 63: 1186–1198
34. Kelly PJ, Alker GJ (1980) A method for stereotactic laser microsurgery in the treatment of deep seated CNS neoplasms. Appl Neurophysiol 43: 210–215
35. Kelly PJ, Alker GJ (1981) A stereotactic approach to deep-seated central nervous system. Surg Neurol 15: 331–335
36. Kelly PJ, Alker GJ, Goerss S (1982) Computer assisted stereotactic laser microsurgery for the treatment of intracranial neoplasms. Neurosurgery 10: 324–331
37. Kelly PJ, Kall B, Goerss S, Alker GJ (1983) Precision resection of intraaxial CNS lesions by CT-based stereotactic craniotomy and computer monitored CO_2 laser. Acta Neurochir (Wien) 68: 1–9

38. Kelly PJ, Kall BA, Goerss SJ (1984) Transposition of volumetric information derived from computed tomography scanning into stereotactic space. Surg Neurol 21: 465–471
39. Kelly PJ, Alker GJ, Kall B, Goerss S (1984) Method of computed-tomography based stereotactic biopsy with arteriographic control. Neurosurgery 14: 172–177
40. Kelly PJ, Kall BA, Goerss S, Earnest F (1985) Present and future developments of stereotactic technology. Appl Neurophysiol 48: 1–6
41. Kelly PJ, Earnest F, Kall BA (1986) Surgical options for patients with deep-seated brain tumours: computer-assisted stereotactic biopsy. Mayo Clin Proc 6: 223–229
42. Kosugi Y, Watanabe E, Goto J, Watanabe T, Yoshimoto S, Takakura K, Ikebe J (1988) An articulated neurosurgical navigation system using MRI and CT images. IEEE Trans Biomed Eng 35: 147–152
43. Kwoh YS, Reed IS, Chen JY, Shao HM, Truong TK, Jonckheere EA (1985) New computerized tomographic-aided robotic stereotaxis system. Robotics Age 7: 17–22
44. Kwoh YS, Hou J, Jonckheere EA, Hayati S (1988) A robot with improved absolute positioning accuracy for CT guided stereotactic brain surgery. IEEE Trans Biomed Eng 35: 153–160
45. Kwoh YS, Young R (1991) Robotic aided surgery. In: Kelly PJ (ed) Computers in stereotactic neurosurgery. Blackwell Scientific Publication, Cambridge (in press)
46. Lavallée S (1989) Gestes médico-chirurgicaux assistés par ordinateur. Thèse Sciences Mathématiques. Université Joseph Fourier, Grenoble
47. Masuzawa H, Kamitani H, Sator J (1981) Intraoperative application of sector scanning electronic ultrasound in neurosurgery. Neurol Med Chir (Tokyo) 21: 277–285
48. Munari C, Betti O (1989) The stereotactic biopsy of brain lesions: a critical review. In: Broggi G, Gerosa MA (eds) Cerebral gliomas. Elsevier Science Publishers, Amsterdam New York Oxford, pp 179–206
49. Mundinger F, Birg W, Klar M (1978) Computer-assisted stereotactic brain operations by means including computerized axial tomography. Appl Neurophysiol 41: 169–182
50. Nguyen JP, Van Effentere R, Fohanno D, Robert G, Sichez JF, Gardeur D (1980) Méthode pratique de repérage spatial des petites néoformations intracrâniennes à partir des données de la tomo-densito-métrie. Neurochirurgie 26: 333–339
51. Oliver A (1986) Double-headed stereotaxic carrier apparatus for insertion of depth electrodes. J Neurosurg 65: 258–259
52. Ostertag CB, Mennel HD, Kiessling M (1980) Stereotactic biopsy of brain tumours. Surg Neurol 14: 275–283
53. Perry JH, Rosenbaum AE, Junsford LD, Swink CA, Zorub DS (1980) Computed tomography-guided stereotactic surgery; Conception and development of a new stereotactic methodology. Neurosurgery 7: 376–381
54. Peters TM, Clark JA, Oliver A, Marchand EP, Mawko G, Dieumegarde M, Muresan LV (1986) Integrated stereotaxic imaging with CT, MR imaging, and digital subtraction angiography. Radiology 161: 821–826

55. Picard C, Olivier A, Bertrand G (1983) The first human stereotaxic apparatus. The contribution of Aubrey Mussen to the field of stereotaxis. J Neurosurg 59: 673–676
56. Roberts DW, Strohbehn JW, Hatch JH, Murray W, Kettenberger H (1986) A frameless stereotaxic integration of computerized tomographic imaging and the operating microscope. J Neurosurg 65: 545–549
57. Roth ZS, Mooring BW, Ravani B (1987) An overview of robot calibration. IEEE J Rob Automat 3: 377–385
58. Scerrati M, Fiorentino A, Fiorentino M, Pola P (1984) Stereotaxic device for polar approaches in orthogonal systems. Technical note. J Neurosurg 61: 1146–1147
59. Schad L, Lott S, Schmitt F, Sturm V, Lorenz WJ (1987) Correction of spatial distortion in MR imaging: a prerequisite for accurate stereotaxy. J Comput Assist Tomogr 11: 499–505
60. Schaltenbrand G, Wahren W (1977) Atlas for stereotaxy of the human brain, 2nd edition. G Thieme, Stuttgart
61. Sedan R, Duparet R (1968) Stéréomètre adaptable au cadre stéréotaxique de J Talairach. Neurochirurgie 14: 577–582
62. Sedan R, Peragut JC, Farnarier Ph, Vallicioni PA (1987) Imagerie moderne et stéréotaxie. Neurochirurgie 33: 29–32
63. Smets C, Vandermeulen D, Suetens P, Oosterlinck A (1989) A knowledge-based system for the 3 D reconstruction and representation of the cerebral blood vessels from a pair of stereoscopic angiograms. Proceedings SPIE 1092, Medical Imaging III, pp 130–138
64. Spiegel EA, Wycis HT, Marks M, Lee A (1947) Stereotactic apparatus for operations on the human brain. Science 57: 164–167
65. Steinmetz H, Fürst G, Freund HJ (1989) Cerebral cortical localization: application and validation of the proportional grid system in MR imaging. J Comput Assist Tomogr 13: 10–19
66. Suetens P, Jansen P (1983) 3 D reconstruction of the blood vessels of the brain from a stereoscopic pair of substraction angiograms. Image and vision computing 1: 43–51
67. Szikla G, Peragut JC (1975) Irradiation interstitielle des gliomes. In: Constans JP, Schlienger M (eds) Radiothérapie des tumeurs du système nerveux central. Neurochirurgie [Suppl] 21: 187–228, Masson, Paris
68. Szikla G, Bouvier G, Hori T (1975) Localization of brain sulci and convolutions by arteriography. A stereotactic anatomo-radiological study. Brain Res 95: 497–502
69. Szikla G, Bouvier F, Hori T, Petrov V (1977) Angiography of the human brain cortex. Springer, Berlin Heidelberg New York
70. Taren J,Guiot G, Derome P, Trigo JC (1968) Hazards of stereotaxic thalamotomy. Added safety factors in corroborating X-ray target localization with neurophysiological methods. J Neurosurg 29: 173–182
71. Talairach J, Ajuriaguerra J de, David M (1950) A propos des coagulations thérapeutiques sous-corticales. Étude topographique du système ventriculaire en fonction des noyaux gris centraux. Presse Méd 58: 697–701

72. Talairach J, Ajuriaguerra J de, David M (1952) Études steréotaxiques des structures encéphaliques profondes chez l'homme. Technique, intérêt physiologique et thérapeutique. Presse Méd 60: 605–609
73. Talairach J, David M, Tournoux P, Corredor H, Kvasina T (1957) Atlas d'anatomie stéreotaxique des noyaux gris centraux. Masson, Paris
74. Talairach J, Szikla G, Tournoux P, Prossolentis A, Bordas-Ferrer M, Covello L, Jacob M, Mempel E (1967) Atlas d'anatomie stereotaxique du télencéphale. Masson, Paris
75. Tasker RR, Organ LW, Hawrylyshyn P (1982) Investigation on the surgical target for alleviation of involuntary movement disorders. Appl Neurophysiol 45: 261–274
76. Tsutsumi Y, Andoh Y, Inoue N (1982) Ultrasound-guided echo biopsy for deep-seated brain tumours. J Neurosurg 57: 164–167
77. Venaille C, Mischler D, Coatrieux JL, Catros JY (1989) Reconstruction 3 D de reseaux vasculaires en angiographie. Proc. 7° Congress AFCET-RFIA, Paris, pp 1533–1547
78. Vidal P, Hache JC, Hayat S, Guerrouad A, Ben Gayed M, Lepers B (1988) Un microtélémanipulateur chirurgical applicable en neurologie et en ophtalmologie. Congrès IIRIAM, Marseille. Productique Hospitalière
79. Wyper DJ, Turner JW, Patterson J, Condon BR, Grossart KWM, Jenkins A, Hadley DM, Rowan JO (1986) Accuracy of stereotactic localisation using MRI and CT. J Neurol Neurosurg Psychiatry 49: 1445–1448
80. Young RJ (1987) Application of robotics to stereotactic neurosurgery. Neurol Res 9: 123–128

Aspects of the Medical Management in Aneurysmal Subarachnoid Hemorrhage

J. P. Castel

Clinique Universitaire de Neurochirurgie, Groupe Hospitalier Pellegrin, Bordeaux (France)

Contents

Introduction

The severity of an aneurysmal subarachnoid hemorrhage (SAH) is not only related to the direct effect of the initial bleeding, but also to the harmful effects of a number of complications occurring in the first two weeks after the ictus. During this time, careful monitoring of the patient and some medical adjuncts can either prevent the occurrence or limit the effects of these complications. Among them, recurrent hemorrhage from the aneurysm and delayed cerebral ischemia are two major events that can dramatically affect the final outcome. Prevention of rebleeding is assured by the surgical exclusion of the aneurysm, whenever possible. Prevention of delayed cerebral ischemia can only be provided by a medical management either pre- or postoperatively. Various drugs have been tried and most of them abandoned becaused of lack of effect. Recent data suggest a role for that calcium antagonists in the prevention of cerebral ischemic complications. Despite early prevention, however, symptoms of cerebral ischemia can occur and a vigorous treatment is needed to reduce the risks of cerebral infarction. The main goal of this treatment has not changed over the years: improvement of cerebral perfusion pressure and thereby of cerebral blood flow.

This chapter documents and discusses some medical aspects of the management of a patient presenting with recent aneurysmal subarachnoid hemorrhage (SAH) and focuses on the complications occurring after SAH such as rebleeding, cardiac arrhythmias, hyponatremia, seizures, and delayed cerebral ischemia associated with vasospasm. All these complications are common, can be diagnosed readily with conventional methods, and a prophylactic or curative treatment is everywhere available. The literature from the past ten years has been reviewed. Deliberately, references are restricted to clinical trials or reports on new treatments proceeding sufficient data. Experimental studies are cited only when they appear to elucidate discussion or controversy.

Prevention of Rebleeding

Recurrent hemorrhage is a major complication generally occurring during the first two weeks after aneurysmal subarachnoid hemorrhage. Often fatal, recurrent bleeding may drastically alter the prognosis for an initially alert patient. Aoyagi and Hayakama (1984) claimed that after a second bleed an alert patient has the same prognosis as a patient admitted in coma after his first hemorrhage. Operative exclusion of the ruptured aneurysm is the best method to prevent recurrence of hemorrhage, but for some patients the optimal time for surgery remains uncertain, depending essentially on their clinical condition. Antifibrinolytic agents have been prescribed to reduce the risk of rebleeding in patients waiting for the operation. Originally, in the course of experimental electrically induced thrombi of the femoral artery of the dog, it was found that one life of thrombi was prolonged, when an antifibrinolytic agent (epsilon-aminocaproïc acid) was previously administered (Mullan *et al.* 1964). It was proposed that antifibrinolytic agents would inhibit the dissolution of blood clot around the fundus of an aneurysm. Since then, antifibrinolytic agents combined with bed rest, sedatives and antihypertensive drugs, have been proved to limit the rate of early rebleeding in patients who are not candidates for early repair of their ruptured intracranial aneurysm. Antifibrinolytic agents interfer with the fibrinolytic activity of the cerebrospinal fluid (CSF), which markedly increases during the first hours after the hemorrhage. Blood present in the CSF activates the conversion of plasminogen to plasmin, inducing the lysis of the clot. Antifibrinolytic agents inhibit this conversion of plasminogen to plasmin and limit the direct effect of plasmin.

I. Drug Administration

Epsilon-aminocaproïc acid (EACA) and tranexamic acid (TEA) are the two antifibrinolytic agents commonly used in SAH. Aminocaproïc acid requires large doses to inhibit fibrinolysis. Oral administration of 24 g to 36 g per day provides the optimal antifibrinolytic effect (Lindsay 1987). Tranexamic acid (6 g/day) should be administered intravenously to promptly provide an adequate serum level of 10 to 15 µg/ml (Fodstad *et al.* 1981). Tranexamic acid is ten times more potent than aminocaproïc acid. Both drugs have the ability to cross the blood-brain barrier. Corroboration of the antifibrinolytic effect of the treatment has been assessed by monitoring either the serum plasminogen concentration level in blood or the fibrin/fibrinogen degradation products in the CSF (Alvarez Garijo *et al.* 1980, Maurice-Williams *et al.* (1980), Fodstad *et al.* 1981, Sawaya *et al.* 1983, Burchiel *et al.* 1984, Vermeulen *et al.* 1985). In some patients who failed to respond to therapy, the recurrence of rebleeding was found to be correlated with a residual high plasminogen activity in the plasma (Burchiel *et al.* 1984), or high levels of fibrin/fibrinogen degradation product (FDP) in CSF at or above 16 µg/ml (Sawaya *et al.* 1983). However, the role of FDP in CSF in monitoring the antifibrinolytic activity was denied by Vermeulen *et al.* (1985). They measured FDP, plasminogen and total protein in the CSF of 48 patients who formed part of a multicentric trial on TEA. Despite the reduction in the incidence of rebleeding in patients treated with TEA, no difference in FDP levels was found in the CSF of patients randomly assigned to TEA treatment compared to the group of patients receiving placebo (Vermeulen *et al.* 1985). These authors suggested that "the presence of FDP's in the CSF reflects a damaged blood-CSF barrier rather than ongoing local fibrinolysis in the subarachnoid space".

II. Results of the Treatment

Almost simultaneously, Mullan and Dawley (1968) and Norlen and Thulin (1969) published the first clinical experience of antifibrinolytic therapy in aneurysmal SAH. These preliminary results were confirmed in a large series of 502 patients who had their proven rebleed rate reduced to 12.7% (Nibbelink *et al.* 1975). Since then, many favourable reports confirmed the favourable effect of antifibrinolytics in reducing the incidence of rebleeding.

Reviewing carefully the results of 25 published series, however, Ramirez-Lassepas (1981) did not accredit this general favourable opinion. Except in 1 out of 12, all the non-controlled studies were favourable to the drug, documenting reduction of the rate of rebleeding, whereas mortality seemed uninfluenced by the treatment. By contrast, no effect of the treatment either on rebleeding or mortality rate was found in 6 of the 13 controlled trials. In two of these studies, recurrence of hemorrhage was twice that of controls, and in all of these studies except one the mortality figures were greater in the treated patients. Similarly, Lindsay (1987) also reviewed 14 uncontrolled studies and confirmed that all authors save one reported favourable results in which rebleeding rates ranged from 0% to 17.8%. In these studies the number of patients included varied from 4 to 1114. Among 17 controlled randomized or non-randomized studies, Lindsay (1987) showed that statistically significant reduction of rebleeding was associated with antifibrinolytic therapy in only six studies, mortality of the patients treated being significantly reduced in only two series. These results are disappointing: despite a potential role of antifibrinolytic therapy to prevent rebleeding, the mortality after aneurysmal SAH was not substantially reduced. In two large series (Kassell *et al.* 1984, Vermeulen *et al.* 1984), it was clearly demonstrated that, whereas the incidence of rebleed and mortality from rebleed were reduced by antifibrinolytic therapy, there was a dramatic concommitant increase in the incidence of cerebral ischemia and death due to cerebral infarction (see Table 1). In the International Cooperative Study on Timing of Aneurysmal Surgery, 672 patients were scheduled for delayed surgery, and 467 of them received EACA or TEA (Kassell *et al.* 1984). The rebleeding rate and the mortality from rebleeding were respectively

Table 1. *Comparative Results of the Incidence and Death from Rebleeding or from Cerebral Infarction in Patients Treated With or Without Antifibrinolytics* (Kassell *et al.* 1984, Vermeulen *et al.* 1984)

	Kassell *et al.* 1984		Vermeulen *et al.* 1984	
n Patients	Anti-fibrinolytics 467	No-anti-fibrinolytics 205	Anti-fibrinolytics 241	No-anti-fibrinolytics 238
Incidence of rebleeding	11.7%	19.4%	9.0%	24.0%
Death from rebleeding	24.0%	45.0%	23.0%	51.0%
Incidence of cerebral infarction	32.4%	22.7%	24.0%	15.0%
Death from cerebral infarction	42.0%	24.0%	45.0%	27.0%

reduced by 39% and 46%. In the Dutch multicenter placebo-controlled randomized study, 479 patients were included and 241 were assigned to TEA treatment (Vermeulen *et al.* 1984). The rebleeding rate and the mortality from rebleeding were respectively reduced by 62% and 54%. Curiously, the death from rebleeding or from cerebral infarction was quite similar in both studies (see Table 1).

III. Complications of the Treatment

Complications due to treatment can occur during the period of the antifibrinolytic treatment with EACA or TEA. Some of these complications include:

— Antifibrinolytics can interfere with blood coagulation and may lead to increased venous thrombosis or pulmonary embolism. However, thromboembolic complications were not markedly increased in a series of 1114 patients analysed by Adams *et al.* 1981. Superficial venous thrombosis occurred in 4,7% of the patients, deep venous thrombosis in 1.2% and pulmonary embolism in 0.7% of the patients.

— Diarrhea and nausea were the commonest unpleasant gastro-intestinal symptoms reported (Adams *et al.* 1981), occurring in half of the patients treated with tranexamic acid.

— All patients receiving more than 24 g per day of aminocaproïc acid have their bleeding time prolonged ranging from 9 to 20 minutes (Glick *et al.* 1981). In all patients the other coagulation tests were within normal limits. The bleeding time returned to normal range within 48 hours of the end of the treatment.

— An increased incidence of communicating hydrocephalus has been observed with the administration of aminocaproïc acid (Park 1979). In 46 patients receiving EACA, hydrocephalus was observed in 43% of the patients and was clinically apparent in 31%. Conversely, in 48 patients not receiving the drug, hydrocephalus was present in only 17% of them, being symptomatic in 10%. This increase in the rate of hydrocephalus was confirmed in other studies but did not reach a significant statistical level (Kassell *et al.* 1984, Vermeulen *et al.* 1984). The production mechanism of cisternal blockade leading to hydrocephalus is still controversial but could be due to the loss of natural fibrinolysis due stopped by the action of EACA.

— Proximal limb and truncal myopathy has been reported on several occasions. Myopathy could be considered as a common complication of prolonged use of antifibrinolytic therapy, especially in patients receiving the treatment for more than 2 weeks and a total dose of greater than 500 g (Brown *et al.* 1982). Muscle biopsy at the onset of the symptoms has shown a necrotizing myopathy, suggested as due to intravascular coagulation or a direct effect of EACA acting as a lysine analogue on the sarcolemna.

— Experimental intravenous or intracisternal administration of aminocaproïc acid in cats resulted in extreme epileptiform changes in the electroencephalogram, and a marked rise in intracranial pressure and blood pressure (Yamaura *et al.* 1980). These experimental findings appeared to be a direct toxic effect of the drug not related to antifibrinolytic activity of the drug.

— Antifibrinolytic treatment undoubtedly increases the risk of cerebral ischemia (Fodstad *et al.* 1978, Ameen *et al.* 1981, Fodstad *et al.* 1981, Fodstad 1982, Kassell *et al.* 1984, Vermeulen *et al.* 1984). As the development of vasospasm is related to the persistence of blood in the CSF, it has been suggested that clearance of blood clots from around the cisterns is delayed by antifibrinolytics, thus leading to a prolonged exposure of the vessels to vasospastic substances. Furthermore, cerebral blood flow was significantly reduced in patients under tranexamic acid treatment, especially on the side of the ruptured aneurysm (Tsementsis *et al.* 1990). Even when the duration of the treatment has been shortened, no reduction in the rate of ischemic complications was reported in a prospective study carried on 119 patients receiving TEA 6 g/day for a maximum of 96 hours (Wijdicks *et al.* 1989). The incidence of cerebral ischemia and the rate of mortality from cerebral ischemia (see Table 1) were similar in the two largest series of the literature reviewing the effects of antifibrinolytics (Kassell *et al.* 1984, Vermeulen *et al.* 1984).

IV. Conclusion

Weir's conclusion (1987) accords with our own; antifibrinolytics have no place in the standard medical management of aneurysmal SAH. Whenever possible, early surgical exclusion of the ruptured aneurysm is one preferred management in prevention of rebleeding. There is no evidence of a beneficial effect of antifibrinolytic drugs, and there is convincing evidence of a potential increase in the incidence and severity of delayed cerebral ischemia for which there is no definite treatment. However, it must be stressed that there is at present no other medical therapy to prevent of aneurysm rebleeding (Adams 1987), and antifibrinolytic therapy may still be administered to some patients admitted within the first week after SAH who are not candidates for early surgery. The addition of calcium antagonists to TEA treatment has been reported by Beck *et al.* (1988) to limit the incidence of cerebral infarction, although these findings have not yet been confirmed by others.

Prevention and Treatment of Cardiac Arrhythmias

I. Incidence

Electrocardiographic (ECG) abnormalities are frequently seen in patients admitted early after subarachnoid hemorrhage. Rare cardiac arrhythmias may also be evident on admission, and some patients are initially admitted to a cardiological intensive care unit. Electrocardiographic changes associated with subarachnoid hemorrhage are not specific and can be associated with many other acute neurological lesions, trauma, meningitis, tumors or cerebral infarction (Marion *et al.* 1986). Comparing 406 patients with subarachnoid hemorrhage and 400 patients with intracranial tumor, the incidence of ECG abnormalities was significantly higher in subarachnoid hemorrhage (Rudehill *et al.* 1987) and approximated to 80%. A prospective study using ECG Holter monitoring initiated within 48 hours of SAH (Andreoli *et al.* 1987) in 70 patients revealed arrhythmias in 91% (64/70) judged as severe in 41% (29/70).

Cardiac arrhythmias are though to be a major cause of sudden death in the early days after subarachnoid hemorrhage, and indeed fatal arrhythmias have been well documented (Estañol *et al.* 1979). Cardiac arrhythmias may however be a less frequent occurrence than sudden respiratory arrest. Among 254 patients Hijdra *et al.* (1984) examined those who had a sudden loss of consciousness and found that within six hours of the first subarachnoid hemorrhage, 37 presented with respiratory disorders and only two had fatal cardiac arrhythmia. Nevertheless, the role of acute cardiac disease and/or ECG changes in the early mortality or final poor outcome after aneurysmal subarachnoid hemorrhage remains unknown (Hijdra *et al.* 1984, Tabbaa *et al.* 1987, Brouwers *et al.* 1989).

II. The Type of ECG Abnormality

Electrocardiographic abnormalities are either morphological or rhythmic in their nature and can be classified as following (Andreoli *et al.* 1987, Brouwers *et al.* 1989):

1A. Rhythmic ECG Changes: Cardiac Arrhythmias

1. Life-threatening ventricular arrhythmias: "torsade de pointe", ventricular flutter, ventricular fibrillation.
2. Serious ventricular tachyarrhythmias: ventricular premature complexes as defined in Lown classes 4 and 5 (class 4, successive ventricular premature complex [VPC] with couplets or salvo; class 5, ventricular tachycardia or early diastolic VPC).
3. Tachyarrhythmias: paroxysmal atrial fibrillation, supraventricular tachycardia.
4. Bradyarrhythmias: sino-atrial block, atrio-ventricular dissociation, idioventricular rhythm.
5. Nonsignificant arrhythmias: sporadic supraventricular complexes, VPC as defined in Lown classes 1, 2 and 3, sinusal bradycardia, sinusal tachycardia, sinusal arrhythmia.

1B. Morphological ECG Changes

1. Evidence of cardiac ischemia: ischemic S-T segment, ischemic inverted T wave, transient pathological Q wave.
2. Other abnormalities: Q-Tc interval prolongation, prominent U wave, large upright T wave, short P-R, peaked P.

Arrhythmias of groups 1—4 are considered as serious. Among morphological ECG changes, a prolonged Q-Tc interval can predispose to serious cardiac arrhythmias especially when it is associated with hypokalemia, or catecholamine release.

III. Etiology

The causes of morphological ECG changes induced by SAH are not fully understood, and frequently mimic myocardial ischemia without proven anatomical changes. In the most severe cases, however, structural myocardial damage has been documented (Doshi and Neil-Dwyer 1980, Marion *et al.* 1986, Brouwers *et al.* 1989). Elevation of cardiac enzymes occurs after SAH and can only be explained by the presence of such structural myocardial lesions as subendocardial ischemia, small hemorrhages, or necrosis of the myocardium. In experimental SAH, arrhythmias are seen immediately after a sudden elevation of intracranial pressure, whereas chronic intracranial hypertension induces bradycardia and does not produce ventricular arrhythmias. (Estañol *et al.* 1977). Increased serum catecholamine levels have been associated with ECG changes both in animals and man (Marion *et al.* 1986). High levels of catecholamines especially norepinephrine may result in myocardial damage either by elevation of the arterial blood pressure with left ventricular strain or by a direct toxic effect. Experimental data and clinicopathological findings support the hypothesis of structural damage of the hypothalamus as the cause of the increase in sympathetic tone and the "adrenergic storm" in the early hours after subarachnoid hemorrhage (Crompton 1963, Cruickshank *et al.* 1974, Doshi *et al.* 1980). A variety of later symptoms may occur with ECG anomalities such as hypokalemia, and gluco-corticoïd hypersecretion.

IV. Prevention or Treatment

Prophylactic administration of such autonomic blockers as propanolol has been advocated in patients suffering from SAH (Cruickshank *et al.* 1974, Neil-Dwyer *et al.* 1983, Marion *et al.* 1986, Neil-Dwyer *et al.* 1986). In a preliminary study, Cruickshank *et al.* (1975) found that ECG changes occurring in SAH were reversed by the administration of 80 mg of oral propanolol. More recently 51 patients operated on early after their aneurysmal rupture were included in a placebo controlled randomized trial to study the effects of propanolol on the final outcome. In the 23 patients receiving placebo, 11 (47%) had bad outcome at six months, compared with 2 (7%) of the 28 patients assigned to oral propanolol 80 mg, a significant difference. Although these findings are encouraging, it has not yet been demonstrated that acute cardiac arrhythmias, or morphologic ECG abnormalities with or without structural subendocardial lesions contribute significantly to morbidity and mortality in SAH. Prophylactic administration of sympathetic blockers remains controversial(Stober *et al.* 1988).

The clinician must beware of the cardiac symptoms and ECG abnormalities that can occur in SAH, and treat them appropriately. ECG monitoring or frequent intermittent ECG control is strongly recommended in the early days after SAH. In the absence of any previous cardiac dysfunction, the majority of the ECG abnormalities in SAH are detected within 48 hours after the admission. Only cardiac arrhythmias are to be treated vigorously, although extreme caution should be taken in the presence of prolonged Q-T interval. Propanolol may be the more appropriate treatment, and can be administered orally or intravenously, but in excess can induce prolonged and harmful hypotension. Esmolol chlorhydrate, a ß blocker with a quick and brief action, can be infused intravenously in case of supraventricular tachycardias. Long lasting arterial hypotension is less of a risk since stopping the infusion will rapidly reverse any blood pressure fall. In case of serious cardiac arrhythmias, consultant cardiological opinion should be sought preoperatively.

Prevention and Treatment of Hyponatremia

After aneurysmal subarachnoid hemorrhage, hyponatremia occurs with an incidence of 9 to 33% (Doczi *et al.* 1981, Wijdicks *et al.* 1985, Diringer 1988). It is never severe, the lowest serum sodium level reported has been 120 meq/l, and as a rule, the serum sodium concentration fluctuate between 125 and 130 meq/l (Joynt *et al.* 1965, Fox *et al.* 1971, Wise 1978, Takaku *et al.* 1979, Doczi *et al.* 1981, Nelson *et al.* 1981, Wijdicks *et al.* 1985, Weinand *et al.* 1989).

I. Signs and Symptoms

Generally, the first symptoms associated with hyponatremia are nonspecific, consisting of nausea, anorexia, emesis, muscle weakness, lethargy, seizures and confusion (Arieff *et al.* 1976). Patients usually became symptomatic when the serum sodium level was below 125 meq/l, seizures occurring with levels below 121 meq/l, and lethargy or coma occurring when the serum sodium level is below 115 to 118 meq/l. The severity of clinical deterioration is related first to the rapidity with which hyponatremia develops, and secondly to the level of the serum sodium. Symptoms are usually rapidly reversed by adequate rapid treatment.

Hyponatremia can make worse any critical neurological situation, but its exact role in clinical deterioration after aneurysmal subarachnoid hemorrhage has not been clearly documented. In a series of 134 consecutive patients with aneurysmal SAH, 44 patients developed hyponatremia with a serum sodium level below 135 meq/l (Wijdicks *et al.* 1985). Cerebral infarction occurred in 27 of these 44 patients with hyponatremia, while in the remaining 90 patients who did not develop hyponatremia only 19 had cerebral infarction. Twenty-six of the 44 patients with hyponatremia received fluid restriction, and the resulting cerebral infarction was supposed to be due to concomitant hypovolemia in 21 of them. Wijdicks *et al.* (1985) emphasized the harmful effect of dehydration in the management of patients with hyponatremia, and did not regard hyponatremia as the main cause of neurological deterioration. In other clinical reports, the rate of complications associated with hyponatremia has been lower (Diringer *et al.* 1988, Doczi *et al.* 1988, Hasan *et al.* 1989, Rosenfeld *et al.* 1989, Shimoda *et al.* 1989).

II. Etiology

Hyponatremia is associated with an inappropriate degree of natriuresis, and this syndrome has been attributed to an inappropriate secretion of anti-diuretic hormone (Lester and Nelson 1981). The syndrome of inappropriate secretion of antidiuretic hormone (SIADH) was described by Schwartz and Bartter (1957). The diagnostic criteria for SIADH are: hyponatremia < 135 meq/l for at least two consecutive days — serum hypoosmolarity < 280 milliosmoles/kg — urinary sodium concentration > 25 meq/l — hyperosmolar urine — apparent normovolemia without osmodiuretic therapy in the absence of renal, adrenal, thyroid or cardiac disease. SIADH is non-specific and has been reported in various other pathological neurological conditions (Lester and Nelson 1981).

Nelson *et al.* (1981) denied the role of inappropriate secretion of the antidiuretic hormone, as they failed to find consistent elevation in the serum antidiuretic hormone concentration in a series of 12 patients with the required criteria of SIADH (10 patients with subarachnoid hemorrhage, and 2 with head injury). They recalled that in the early 1950's, worsening in the patient's neurological condition associated with hyponatremia was referred to as "cerebral salt wasting" (Cort 1954). This condition is markedly different from SIADH. In the "cerebral salt wasting syndrome" (CSWS), renal salt loss leads to progressive salt and extracellular volume depletion. This is an "inappropriate natriuresis" despite the depressed concentration of sodium in the serum, and hyponatremia is due to excessive salt loss. Conversely, in SIADH, water intoxication leads to an expanded and increased extracellular volume, and hyponatremia is due to serum sodium dilution. CSWS and SIADH should receive quite opposite form of treatment, in the former additional salt supply is necessary with correction of the vascular volume, and in the latter water restriction is the treatment of choice.

The exact cause of this natriuresis remains unknown. Nelson *et al.* (1981) first suggested "a yet undefined natriuretic factor in the brain" that alone or with an alteration of renal innervation might be responsible for the inappropriate natriuresis. Recently, a new peptide, Atrial Natriuretic Factor (ANF), has been described (Goetz 1988, Quirion 1988). ANF is synthesized either in the cardiac ventricles and atria rather than in the brain. There is some evidence that in patients with hyponatremia and excessive natriuresis, serum antidiuretic hormone level remains low (Nelson *et al.* 1984), and concomitantly plasma concentration of ANF is elevated (Diringer *et al.* 1989, Weinand *et al.* 1989). In subarachnoid hemorrhage, ANF in serum is increased two to seven times the normal range (Diringer *et al.* 1988, Diringer *et al.* 1989, Rosenfeld *et al.* 1989, Shimoda *et al.* 1989). This elevation lasts for 8 to 10 days or even more and progressively decreases. The relationship between ANF and natriuresis on the one hand and between ANF and ADH on the other hand are not clearly demonstrated (Diringer *et al.* 1989, Rosenfeld *et al.* 1989, Shimoda *et al.* 1989). It is proposed that a neural modulation of ANF release and the renal effects of ANF are related. At all event the exact role of this "inappropriate secretion of ANF" in the changes in serum electrolytes after SAH remains unclear. If this persistent excess of ANF is documented as the major factor of "cerebral salt-wasting syndrome", then, in the near future, ANF antagonist peptides may be developed to manage the condition.

III. Treatment

Nelson *et al.* (1981) suggested a pragmatic and less complex pathological cascade related to the inapropriate natriuresis: 1. initial progressive loss of sodium leads to volume depletion; 2. volume depletion is a strong stimulus for secretion of ADH; 3. excess in ADH secretion leads to water retention; 4. water retention along with progressive renal loss of sodium leads to hyponatremia. This may explain why some patients with aneurysmal subarachnoid hemorrhage and precessive adequate or inadequate medical management present with such a variety of electrolytic conditions associated to hyponatremia.

Correction of hyponatremia may require both fluid restriction, salt supplements and correction of hypovolemia. Fluid restriction should be avoided as the major treatment of hyponatremia in subarachnoid hemorrhage, leading consistently to hypovolemia and subsequent cerebral ischemia (Wijdicks *et al.* 1985). Furthermore, fluid restriction is too slow in the correction of hyponatremia, and it is difficult to apply in patients requiring intravenous fluid intake for medication or parenteral nutrition. On the contrary, correction of hypovolemia is essential in the management of hyponatremia. With the infusion of colloids, particularly balanced salt solutions, hypovolemic dehydration and hyponatremia can simultaneously be corrected. Additionally, daily fluid intake should be kept higher than 2000 ml given either orally or intravenously (isotonic saline).

Increase in sodium intake can be provided either by oral or intravenous administration of sodium chloride. Oral prescription is commonly used, if needs be through a nasogastric tube in a comatose patient. Intravenous intake is limited by the fact that only isotonic solutions are accepted, hypertonic saline should only be used in severe cases when serum sodium level is below 115 mosml. To avoid serious necrotizing effects on the peripheral veins, hypertonic solution should be administered via a central venous catheter. To limit the renal sodium loss, low doses of salidiuretics have been used but this can lead to a dangerous increase in salt wasting and uncontrolled dehydration. Decaux *et al.* (1982) advocated the use of urea and increased sodium intake as an alternative to the urgent correction of hyponatremia in SIADH. Reeder and Harbaugh (1989) reported their favourable clinical experience in 48 patients. This treatment was started when the serum sodium level dropped to 132 mmol or less, with an intravenous injection of 40 mg of urea in 100 or 150 milliliters of isotonic saline. Isotonic saline 60 to 100 ml/hour was then infused intravenously, urea infusion repeated every 48 hours. With this treatment, correction of hyponatremia occurs likely within 24 hours.

Prevention of hyponatremia is achieved with control of the sodium and fluid balance. Fludrocortisone has been recommended in the prevention of a negative sodium balance (excessive natriuresis) associated with a negative fluid balance and a plasma volume depletion (Hasan *et al.* 1989). In a randomized multicenter trial, it was found that fludrocortisone administered to 46 of 91 patients with SAH significantly reduced the natriuresis during the first 6 days. The reduction of negative sodium balance resulting from the fludrocortisone administration tended to limit the decrease in plasma volume, although the difference was not statistically significant (Hasan *et al.* 1989). Fludrocortisone was administered intravenously or orally, 400 μg/day in divided doses, for a maximum duration of 12 days. During the treatment, fluid intake was maintained at 3 liters per day either orally or intravenously.

Should hyponatremia always be vigorously corrected or not? The answer is no when hyponatremia is found in the first days after SAH. It may be due to a previous renal or hormonal dysregulation, and is well tolerated. The answer is again no in the absence of specific neurological symptoms[1]. Hyponatremia occurring during the first week after an aneurysmal subarachnoid hemorrhage should be considered as a symptom of nonspecific dysregulation of sodium balance. Nevertheless, the serum sodium concentration should be assessed thoroughly during the first 10 days post-SAH. If the serum sodium level decreases below 122 to 125 meq/l, or if any neurological deterioration occurs, then hyponatremia should be promptly corrected.

Prevention of Seizures and Epilepsy

Epileptic seizures can occur after aneurysmal SAH, either at the onset of the hemorrhage, or later during the postoperative period. The overall incidence of epileptic seizures after SAH is reported to range between 10 to 26% of the patients (Hart *et al.* 1981). The aim of prophylactic treatment with anticonvulsants is to prevent maturation of the epileptic focus or to prevent early or delayed recurrence of the fits. However, the value of preventive anticonvulsant therapy given to patients with aneurysmal subarachnoid hemorrhage is uncertain, mainly because the seizures occurring after SAH are related to different etiological mechanisms depending on the time of their occurrence. Seizures occurring early after the initial hemorrhage (at the onset or within the first 24 hours or days after SAH) are considered as an epiphenomenon of the acute brain stress following the aneurysm bleeding. Conventionally, they are designated as "early seizures". Seizures, especially recurrent seizures occurring one month or later after SAH, are considered the clinical expression of permanent brain damage with an epileptic focus, and are properly described as "late epilepsy".

I. Early Seizures

"Early seizures" occur within hours or days after the initial hemorrhage. They occurred at the onset of the hemorrhage, in a recent prospective study, in 19% of the patients (Hart *et al.* 1981). The seizures are usually brief and generalized accompanied by loss of consciousness and incontinence. Status epilepticus rarely occurs. Twenty percent of recurrent bleeding episodes were associated with seizures within 12 hours (Hart *et al.* 1981). The findings support the view that hemorrhage induces the epileptic activity. Early seizures do not indicate a likelihood of late epilepsy, and are not useful predictors of outcome, except in their tight relationship with recurrent hemorrhage.

Prophylactic treatment of "early seizures" remains controversial because of their low incidence, and their relationship with rebleeding episodes. Nevertheless, a patient presenting with early seizures should be given anticonvulsants, at least transiently, even if only to prevent early recurrence of the fits. A rapid serum concentration level consistent with clinical efficiency is best achieved with intravenous administration. Traditionally, intravenous phenytoin 250 mg twice a day is administered initially, with a further oral prescription of 100 mg three times a day. Clonazepam 1 mg to 2 mg/day, a benzodiazepine derivative, can be infused intravenously, after a direct intravenous injection of a 0.5 mg to 1 mg loading dose. Clonazepam is as effective as phenytoin, with possibly less adverse effects.

II. Late Epilepsy

A patient presenting seizures one month or more after the aneurysm rupture, whereas apparently stable after his operation, is a risk of post-SAH "late epilepsy". From the combined results of five large series of aneurysms operated (a total of 1772 patients), the rate of postoperative epilepsy ranged between 1% and 7% (Sbeih *et al.* 1986). In another series of 177 patients operated on for a ruptured aneurysm, late seizures occurred in 14% (25/177), and seizures were recurrent in 12% (21/177) (Keränen *et al.* 1985). In their personal series of 100 patients who survived their aneurysm operation, Sbeih *et al.* (1986) found only 3 patients who developed late epilepsy and stated that the risk of postoperative epilepsy seemed to have declined, perhaps as the result of technical improvement in the microsurgical approach and anesthetic management. In conservatively treated patients with cerebral aneurysms, Winn *et al.* (1978) found seizure disorders in less than 10% of the patients.

Some risk factors have been identified for postoperative epilepsy after aneurysm clipping: presence of an intracerebral hematoma, large brain resection, prolonged medial temporal retraction, persistent major postoperative deficit. All these factors indicate permanent parenchymal brain damage evolving toward an epileptic focus. Aneurysms located on the middle cerebral artery have also been shown to carry a higher risk of late epilepsy than other aneurysmal locations. Chronic alcoholism is another factor of risk, from the lower epileptic threshold in such patients. Additionally, craniotomy and surgical exposure may combine their effects with the initial cerebral lesion associated with the subarachnoid hemorrhage in the production of brain damage to a possible late focus.

Double-blind trials on phenytoin prophylaxis either in head injury or in craniotomies failed to show an effect in preventing epilepsy (North *et al.* 1983, Young *et al.* 1983). The overall incidence of late epilepsy after aneurysmal SAH or after craniotomy is extremely low, making difficult valid conclusions about the lack of effect of a prophylactic drug different. More than 90% of the patients have a low risk profile for "late epilepsy". So, the low incidence of late epilepsy after SAH should be stressed more than the hypothetical benefit of prophylaxis and the use of an undue and long-lasting prescription of anticonvulsants abandoned.

After aneurysm operation, prophylactic anticonvulsants should be given only to patients who are at a high risk of developing late epilepsy. The following scale is indicative: a patient who accumulates more than 5 to 6 points should have anticonvulsant prophylaxis.

Permanent neurological deficit	4 points
Intracerebral hemorrhage	3 points
Prolonged unconsciousness (> 2 weeks)	2 points

Multiple cerebral infarcts	2 points
Surgical brain trauma or resection	1 point
Middle cerebral artery Aneurysm	1 point
Chronic alcoholism	1 point

Prevention of Cerebral Arterial Vasospasm

According to Wilkins (1986), cerebral arterial vasospasm after SAH is categorised by 1. an angiographically evident focal or diffuse narrowing of the lumen of the major intracranial arteries; 2. a delayed neurological deterioration thought to be due to cerebral ischemia; 3. the combination of arterial vasospasm and the symptoms of a delayed cerebral ischemia. The aim of a prophylaxis is to prevent the development of the arterial narrowing and to decrease the risk of cerebral ischemia or to limit the extension of subsequent cerebral infarction. The pathogenesis of cerebral vasospasm is not yet clearly understood. The release of vasoactive substances from the subarachnoid clot is thought to be one of the major factor of the arterial narrowing. Recently attention has been focused on the participation of arterial endothelial damage to the persistent cerebral arterial narrowing with the subsequent effects on the cerebral circulation (Kassell *et al.* 1985, Bevan and Bevan 1988). Furthermore, the reduction in the circulating blood volume which spontaneously occurs in patients after SAH, can proportionally impair the cerebral circulation.

Prevention of cerebral vasospasm can be attempted by restoring or elevating the circulating blood volume and by the early administration of specific drugs. Specific drugs to protect from cerebral ischemia are still under experimental research, but many agents have been tested in clinical practice to prevent or to limit the extension of arterial constriction (Wilkins 1986). Since the 80's, the use of calcium antagonists has been proposed with both experimental and clinical support, and special clinical interest has been focussed on nimodipine.

I. Correction of Hypovolemia

A. Incidence

Hypovolemia occurs spontaneously in patients presenting with aneurysmal subarachnoid hemorrhage. This decrease in total blood volume (i.e., red cell volume + plasma volume) was first measured in patients by Maroon and Nelson (1979), using radio-isotope labeled erythrocytes and albumin. In a series of 15 patients, they found that the total blood volume was reduced by 17%, equivalent to 850 milliliters loss of blood volume in a patient weighting 70 kilograms. Hypovolemia in SAH was confirmed later by Solomon *et al.* (1984) in 35 patients. An abnormally low total blood volume and a relative deficit of the red blood cells volume affected respectively 46% and 65% of the patients, and females presented more frequently with hypovolemia.

B. Etiology

The exact cause of hypovolemia in SAH remains unknown and may well be multifactorial. In a normal individual, prolonged bed rest is associated after 10 days with decreased in the red cell volume of 140 to 215 ml. At the same time, plasma volume can be decreased as much as 500 ml. Excess fluid loss (due to hyperthermia, vomiting, enhanced natriuresis, diuretics) associated with decrease in fluid intake (fluid restriction, gastric intolerance, prolonged fasting) contribute to hypovolemia. Daily blood loss for sampling, and elevation of the head of the bed are also contributory factors.

Hypovolemia is considered as an important factor contributing to the development of cerebral ischemia in the presence of vasospasm (Maroon and Nelson 1979, Solomon *et al.* 1984, Wijdicks *et al.* 1985, Wilkins 1986). In a group of 46 patients, an increase in the daily fluid intake (minimum 3 l per day) significantly decreased the occurrence of cerebral ischemia after SAH compared with a group of patients treated with fluid restriction (Hasan *et al.* 1989). When cerebral autoregulation is intact, cerebral blood flow (CBF) is relatively independent of physiological variations in perfusion pressure. If autoregulation is altered as it is in SAH, then CBF becomes dependent on systemic hemodynamic conditions. In animal experiments, staged hypovolemia without arterial hypotension caused successive decrements in cardiac output and CBF (Davis and Sundt 1980). At the end of the procedure, the cardiac output was reduced by 32% and the CBF by 24%. This can be termed "a coupled response of cardiac output and CBF to hypovolemia" (Yamakami *et al.* 1987). In the presence of intact autoregulation, CBF was not increased by the elevation of cardiac output (Davis and Sundt 1980). Excess use of antihypertensive drugs with hypovolemia will further lower cerebral perfusion pressure and thereby critically decrease the CBF.

C. Diagnosis and Treatment

The diagnosis of hypovolemia is not easy to confirm. A blood pressure is not an early indicator of hypovolemia. Changes in hematocrit and hemoglobin are not immediately present. Isotopic measurement of the total blood volume is the best way to confirm depletion of the circulating blood volume, but this procedure is not widely available. Measurement of central venous pressure via an intravenous catheter is generally used to estimate the volume of the circulating blood. Normally, the central venous pressure averages of 5 to 6 mmHg, and volume correction should be achieved when central venous pressure maintains this normal level. However, patients can frequently be managed without central venous pressure monitoring. With the patient in a recumbent position, careful appraisal of the volume of visible veins on the limbs or the external jugular veins can give an approximate indication of changes in the central venous pressure.

Overcorrection of hypovolemia leads to hemodilution, a condition that is not always beneficial for the brain circulation (Hino *et al.* 1989). However, an experimental study has suggested that decrease in blood viscosity accounted directly for a favorable increase in cardiac output and CBF after volume expansion by plasma infusion (Wood *et al.* 1984). After SAH, impaired cerebrovascular resistance and impairment of the blood-brain barrier may lead to brain edema, increased intracranial pressure and thereby further reduction of the cerebral perfusion pressure (Voldby *et al.* 1985). Prophylactic hypertensive hypervolemia has been proposed by Solomon *et al.* (1988) to reduce the postoperative incidence of delayed cerebral ischemia after early surgery. Fifty-six consecutive patients were successfully treated with prophylactic volume expansion therapy and hypertension for 14 days, with a central venous pressure or a Swan-Ganz catheter. Ten patients (18%) had delayed cerebral ischemia resulting in 3 permanent deficits and 1 death. A single case of hemorrhagic shock with cardiac arrest due to an inadvertant disconnection of the central venous catheter was reported as the only complication of the treatment. Tanabe *et al.* (1988) studied the prophylactic effect of hypervolemic therapy without hypertension in the postoperative period, and found a 75% reduction of the incidence of cerebral ischemia.

All patients during the first two weeks after their SAH can develop spontaneous hypovolemia. Correction of this hypovolemia should be carried out as early as possible to be effective in prevention of ischemic complications from the cerebral vasospasm. Overcorrection of the hypovolemia can be harmful. In the standard management of SAH, dehydration from fluid restriction or diuretic administration should be discarded and a normal fluid intake should be maintained up to 2 l per day, either orally or intravenously. In addition, the use of antihypertensive drugs to control arterial hypertension must be extremely careful. The control of central venous pressure is virtually essential to achieve perfect volume correction.

II. Calcium Antagonists

A. Pharmacology

The therapeutic value of calcium antagonists was discovered in 1963 and their complete history has been reviewed by Fleckenstein (1983) who is regarded as the "father" of calcium antagonists. Calcium antagonists can affect the movement and the binding of calcium. Calcium antagonists decrease the transmembranal influx of Ca^{++} during Phase 2 depolarization of the cell membrane. Thus, the amount of intracellular Ca^{++} available for activation is restricted. Ca^{++} channels (or V.O.C. for voltage operated channel) are voltage dependent. Among the three classes of VOC described (T for Transient or fast, L for Late or slow, N for Neuronal), only the opened type L channels are affected by calcium antagonists. The most prominent hemodynamic action or the calcium antagonists is to lower the arterial blood pressure in reducing the systemic vascular resistance. A common pharmacokinetic characteristic of all calcium antagonists is an extensive first pass hepatic extraction after oral administration, a high clearance, and an extensive binding to plasma proteins. With a such high clearance (half-lives are 2 or 5 hours), multiple daily doses are required to achieve a steady state plasma concentration (Abenerthy and Schwartz 1988).

The pharmacological effect of a calcium antagonist depends on its selectivity for different tissue slow channels. Using the classification proposed by Singh (1986), calcium antagonists can be classified as Type I drugs that include phenylalkylamines (as verapamil) and benzothiazepines (as diltiazem) and their structural analogues, and Type II drugs that comprise the phenyldihydropyridines as nifedipine and its structural analogues nimodipine, or nicardipine. Calcium antagonists have more affinity with some site or other. Type II drugs are potent peripheral arterial dilators with less negative inotropic effects than Type I drugs. Among dihydropyridines, special attention has been focused on the selectivity of nimodipine for the cerebral arteries, which was higher than that of nifedipine or nicardipine (Kazda 1985).

B. Nimodipine

Nimodipine is a lipid-soluble 1,4-dihydropyridine derivative with cerebrovascular selectivity demonstrated in isolated vessels and in experiments on intact animals (Kazda and Towart 1981). Nimodipine can pass the blood-brain barrier and selectively block the influx of calcium to cerebrovascular smooth-muscle cells. Nimodipine can be administered either by intravenous or oral route. For intravenous infusion, nimodipine is presented in vials containing 10 mg in 50 ml with a special poly-ethylene catheter for the intravenous injection. The vehicle contains 23.7 volume percent of alcohol (10 g in a 50 ml solution). Intravenous recommended dosage is 2 mg/hour. Oral nimodipine is available in tablets containing 30 mg. The oral recommended dosage is 60 mg or 2 tablets every four hours. Pharmacokinetics of the drug have been studied either in volunteers and in patients (Rämsch *et al.* 1985, Vinge *et al.* 1988). Mean serum concentration is expected to average 27 ± 2 ng/ml after 8 hours of intravenous infusion. One hour after each oral dose, the peak plasma concentration averaged 13.2 ng/ml. In some clinical trial, nimodipine serum level concentration has been assessed (Allen *et al.* 1983, Auer 1984, Säveland *et al.* 1986). No major side effects have been reported with the use of nimodipine. The presence of large amounts of alcohol in the vehicle has been criticized, but no direct side effects have been documented. To avoid any arterial hypotension at the onset of the treatment, it is recommended to monitor and correct the patient's blood circulating volume. The duration of the treatment is usually 14 to 21 days. The treatment with intravenous nimodipine 2 mg/hour costs approximately 110 Francs per day (or 16–18 US Dollars).

Harper *et al.* (1981) reported the effect of nimodipine on the cerebral circulation in primate where continuous intravenous infusion of 2 μg/kg/min of nimodipine caused a modest fall in the mean arterial pressure and gradually increased cerebral blood flow by 27% with no significant effect on cerebral metabolism. These experimental findings were largely confirmed later, indicating nimodipine as possibly the ideal drug in case of cerebral ischemia or arterial spasm. Allen *et al.* (1983) reported the results of nimodipine in the prevention of cerebral arterial spasm in patients with subarachnoid hemorrhage. In this study the first multicentre placebo controlled randomized clinical trial on nimodipine, of a total group of 125 patients, 56 patients received orally 20 to 30 mg of nimodipine every four hours, 60 patients were given placebo and 9 patients were excluded from the analysis for protocol violations. Cerebral ischemia occurred in 13 patients treated with nimodipine, and in 16 patients in the placebo group. At the end of the treatment 5 severe neurological deficits and 3 deaths occurred in the 60 patients given placebo, but only one death attributed to cerebral ischemia in the 56 given nimodipine. This study has been criticized because of lack of data concerning final outcome, the surgical procedure, however the rate of non-ischemic complications. Following these favourable preliminary results, clinical trials of nimodipine have been carried out in some European centers, well-known for their expertise in aneurysmal surgery. Most of these prospective studies were "uncontrolled" offering no comparison with a group of patients who did not received the drug (see Table 2). In other "controlled" studies, patients were randomly assigned to the drug or to a placebo (see Table 3). All the important published trials on nimodipine will now be summarized as briefly as possible (see also Tables 2 and 3).

1. Uncontrolled Prospective Studies

1-a) Uncontrolled Single Centre Studies

Auer (1983) reported a short series of 31 patients operated only early and prophylactically treated with intravenous (1 to 2 mg/hour) and then oral

(4 x 60 mg per day) nimodipine. No ischemic complication occurred postoperatively. In 6 cases (19%), unfavourable results were attributed to surgical complications.

Auer (1984) selected 65 patients out of 97 for early surgery. Nimodipine treatment was administered intravenously (1–2-mg/hour) and then orally (4 x 60 mg per day). Postoperative complications occurred in 28 patients and were attributed to reversible or irreversible delayed ischemic symptoms in 4 cases (6.1%) and to surgical complications in 10 patients (15.3%). The conclusion was that nimodipine reduced the management complications and improved the outcome, especially reducing ischemic lesions from symptomatic vasospasm.

Ljunggren *et al.* (1984) presented postoperative results in a series of 60 patients grade 1 to 3 (Hunt and Hess). All patients were operated on early and received prophylactic nimodopine intravenously (2 mg/hour) and then orally (60 mg every four hours). Delayed ischemic deterioration attributable to vasospasm occurred in two patients (3.3%) with one fair outcome and one death. Recovery was uneventful in 78.3% of patients and no surgical complications were reported. The conclusion was that early surgery is beneficial in patients in good clinical condition and that there is an indication that nimodipine provided an additional anti-ischemic effect.

Säveland *et al.* (1986) analyzed 100 consecutive patients admitted early (85 in grades 1 to 3 of Hunt and Hess, and 15 grade 4 or 5), and treated with intravenous nimodipine 2 mg/hour for ten days after early operation. The incidence of delayed ischemic deficit was 7%, transient in 2 cases, permanent in 2 cases, and fatal in 3 cases. It was concluded that nimodipine added good protection against delayed ischemic deterioration.

Seiler *et al.* (1988) treated consecutively 153 patients admitted in all clinical grades within a period of 42 months. All patients were prophylactically treated by intravenous nimodipine 2 mg/hour for 7 to 14 days followed by oral administration of nimodipine 60 mg every four hours for one week. Operation was early in 55 patients and delayed in 57, and 17 patients were not considered for surgery. Delayed ischemic deficit occurred in 8 patients (5.2%) with 6 persistent neurological deficits and 2 deaths.

Hillman *et al.* (1988) in 91 consecutive patients admitted in Hunt and Hess grade 1 to 3 during a 44 months period performed early surgery in 85 of them, and intravenous nimodipine 2 mg/hour was administered pre- or postoperatively for a minimum period of 10 days. The incidence of permanent late ischemic deficit was 3%. Surgical complications occurred in 10 patients (11.7%). They concluded that the low incidence of ischemia suggested a beneficial effect from nimodipine treatment.

Gilsbach and Harders (1989) reported their experience of the treatment with intravenous nimodipine (2 to 3 mg/hour) following early surgery in 116 consecutive patients in good clinical condition (grade 1 to 3 according to Hunt and Hess). The result of treatment was assessed at the end of treatment (2 weeks) and at follow-up. Delayed neurological dysfunction was the cause of morbidity/mortality in 3 patients (3%). However, 13 patients (11%) presented with ischemic neurological deterioration, transient in four. In 7 patients additional complications contributed to exacerbrate vasospasm, and independently from vasospasm, 2 patients had an arterial occlusion considered as the cause of ischemia. Surgical complications occurred in 14 patients (12%). Postoperative computerized tomography revealed cerebral infarction in 24 patients (20.6%), 16 of them being symptomatic. They concluded that in early operation combined with intravenous nimodipine, vasospasm alone is no longer the major clinical problem.

1-b) Uncontrolled Multicentre Studies

Auer *et al.* (1986) reported in a prospective open multicentric study the preventive effect of nimodipine in 120 (consecutive) patients grades 1 to 3 of Hunt and Hess. All patients underwent early surgery. Nimodipine 2 mg/hour was administered intravenously for 7 to 14 days, followed by oral medication (240–270 mg/day) for one more week. Ischemic cerebral dysfunction of delayed onset, associated with a permanent deficit, occurred in 2 patients (2%). In 8 patients (6.7%) transient ischemic deficits were observed. Surgical complications carefully assessed, affected 20 patients (16%) who had some additional neurological deficit immediately after the operation. However, morbidity resulting from intraoperative complications was 5.8% and mortality was 1.7%. The conclusion was that prophylactic nimodipine may reduce delayed ischemic deficit in early aneurysmal surgery.

Gilsbach (1988), in his recent analysis of nimodipine clinical trials, discussed the results of a similar open multicentric study including 237 patients treated with intravenous nimodipine 48 mg/day or 72 mg/day (Gilsbach *et al.* cited as reference 13 in Gilsbach 1988). Exclusions for protocol violations applied to 33 patients. The clinical condition was Hunt and Hess grade 1 to 3 in 162 patients, and grade 4 or 5 in 42 patients. Seven patients (7 of 204 or 3%) suffered ischemic neurological deficit which led to severe disability in 3 patients and death in one patient (1.9% morbidity/mortality). The outcome was not different in the two dosage groups.

2. Placebo-Controlled Randomized Studies

2-a) Controlled Single Centre Studies

Philipon *et al.* (1986) studied a group of 81 patients admitted within 72 hours after their aneurysmal SAH, and presenting in Hunt and Hess grade 1 to 3. Nimodipine 60 mg was administered orally every four hours. Thirty-

Table 2. *Nimodipine in the Prevention of Cerebral Arterial Vasospasm: Uncontrolled Studies*

		n patients	Grade	Timing of Operation	Incidence of severe ischemic deficit	Total morbidity	Total mortality
Unicentre open studies							
Auer	1983	31	1–3	early	0.0%	18.5%	0.0%
Auer	1984	65	1–3	early	6.1%	13.8%	10.7%
Ljunggren *et al.*	1984	60	1–5	early	3.3%	22.0%	1.5%
Säveland *et al.*	1986	100	1–5	early	7.0%	22.0%	7.0%
Seiler *et al.*	1988	153	1–5	early + late	5.2%	14.0%	27.0%
Hillman *et al.*	1988	91	1–3	early	3.0%	?	?
Gilsbach and Harders	1989	116	1–3	early	3.0%	6.8%	10.3%
Multicentre open studies							
Auer *et al.*	1986	120	1–3	early	2.0%	6.6%	2.5%
Gilsbach *et al.*	1988	237	1–5	early	3.0%	6.8%	7.8%

Table 3. *Nimodipine in the Prevention of Cerebral Arterial Vasospasm: Controlled Studies*

		n patients	Exclusions	Grade	Timing of operation	Incidence of severe ischemic deficit		Total morbidity	Total mortality
						Nimodipine	Placebo		
Unicentre controlled studies									
Philippon *et al.*	1986	81	11	1–3	>Day 4	10.0%	33.0%	?	?
Mee *et al.*	1988	75	25	1–5	Late	12.0%	20.0%	16.0%	19.0%
Öhman and Heiskanen	1988	215	2	1–3	1st week	0.0%	11.0%	7.0%	12.0%
Multicentre controlled studies									
Allen *et al.*	1983	125	9	1–3	2–14 days	1.7%	13.3%	?	8.6%
Petruk *et al.*	1988	188	34	3–5	Anytime	6.9%	26.8%	21.0%	43.0%
Pickard *et al.*	1989	554	0	1–5	Anytime	12.0%	18.0%	8.0%	19.0%

one patients were randomly assigned to nimodipine treatment for a 21-day period, 39 were given placebo, and 11 were secondarily excluded for protocol violations. Antifibrinolytics (tranexamic acid 6 g/day) were generally administered in both groups. Operation after the fourth day was carried out in 68% of the patients. The incidence of neurological deficit was 74.4% (29/39) in the placebo group, and 58.1% (18/31) in the nimodipine group. The clinical results were evaluated at the end of the treatment. When the deficit was directly related to vasospasm, it led to bad outcome in 10 patients (25.6%) given placebo (6 severe deficits, 4 deaths), and only in 2 patients (6.4%) given nimodipine (2 deaths). When vasospasm was associated with other complications, the difference in the results were even more significant (13 patients given placebo had severe outcome compared with 3 in the group given nimodipine). The conclusion was that the efficacy of nimodipine in the reduction of the incidence of neurological deficits due to vasospasm was confirmed.

Mee *et al.* (1988) reported the results in 75 consecutive patients of a randomized double-blind placebo-controlled study. Final outcome at 3 months was assessed. Nimodipine 60 mg was given orally every four hours for 21 days. The clinical condition of the patients was judged according to the author's scale (detailed in the text), generally similar to the usual Hunt and Hess grades. Cerebral blood flow was estimated daily using the xenon-133 inhalation method. 25 patients were excluded secondarily, 50 eligible aneurysm patients were included in the main analysis, 25 of them receiving nimodipine and 25 receiving placebo. Operation was performed within 21 days post-SAH in 75% of the patients. Operative complications occurred in 4 nimodipine-treated patients and in 9 placebo-treated patients. Four of the 38 patients given nimodipine died, compared with 10 of the 37 given placebo. From the 50 eligible aneurysm patients, 1 patient (4%) on nimodipine died compared with 6 patients (24%) receiving placebo. The conclusions were that nimodipine did not increase the cerebral blood flow and that the trend toward better outcome should be verified.

Öhman and Heiskanen (1988) reported the effect of intravenous nimodipine in 213 (consecutive?) patients admitted in Hunt and Hess grade 1 to 3 with a ruptured aneurysm. Nimodipine treatment was assigned randomly to 62 patients. Starting the treatment as soon as the diagnosis has been made, nimodipine 2 mg/hour was infused intravenously during 7 to 10 days and then continued for 21 days with oral administration of 60 mg every four hours. Betamethasone 6 x 4 mg was routinely administered. At the final outcome (three months) it was shown that, in patients operated on during the first week, nimodipine significantly decreased the number of deaths due to delayed ischemic deficit, with 1 death (1.6%) in patients given nimodipine, versus 8 deaths (12.3%) in one placebo group.

Öhman and Heiskanen (1989) reported later the results of a placebo-controlled study in 216 patients with 79 patients randomly assigned to nimodipine treatment. In the nimodipine-treated patients, 10 of 79 patients had permanent disability from delayed ischemic deterioration and 1 patient out of 79 died, resulting in a total morbidity plus mortality of 13.9% in that group. Compared to the placebo-treated patients, these results were significantly different ($p < 0.03$). Unfortunately 52 patients were added to the randomly assigned placebo group who did not received nimodipine and who were said to have been managed identically before the nimodipine study started. This addition renders these favorable statistical results difficult to solidate.

2-b) Controlled Multicentre Studies

Petruk *et al.* (1988) reported the results of the Canadian multicentre randomized placebo-controlled trial on nimodipine. The effect of oral nimodipine (90 mg every four hours) was documented in patients admitted in unfavorable grade 3 to 5 of Hunt and Hess within 96 hours after their SAH. Among the 188 patients included, 72 patients received nimodipine and 82 were given placebo; 34 were excluded for protocol violation or statistical considerations. At three months, 21 of the 72 nimodipine-treated patients (29.2%) had good outcome compared to 8 of the 82 placebo-treated patients (9.8%). The mortality rate was higher in the nimodipine group than in the placebo group (47.2% versus 39.0% with no statistical significance), and, without any detectable reason, the largest difference occurred in the patients grade 3 (mortality of 28,0% for nimodipine-treated patients versus 4.8% for placebo-treated patients). Delayed ischemic deficits were observed in 45.8% (33/72) of the patients given nimodipine and in 65.8% (54/82) of those given placebo. Permanent ischemic deficit due to vasospasm alone occurred in 5 nimodipine-treated patients (6.9%) compared to 22 in placebo-treated patients (26.8%). No significant difference in the degree of vasospasm was observed on the second angiogram carried out after day 4 in 124 patients. It was concluded that in poor-grade patients nimodipine increased the number of good outcome and reduced the incidence and severity of delayed ischemic neurological deterioration due to spasm.

Pickard *et al.* (1989) reported the results of the British aneurysm nimodipine trial. The rate of cerebral infarction and the final outcome was studied in 554 patients admitted in all clinical grades within 96 hours of their subarachnoid hemorrhage and randomly assigned to placebo or oral nimodipine 60 mg every four hours for 21 days. The results were assessed at three months after the entry. Only one patient was withdrawn and there was no exclusion after entry. In the 276 placebo-treated patients and in the 278 nimodipine-treated patients, demographic and clinical data at entry were similar. Intracranial aneurysms were present in 66.4% (368/554) of the patients. The incidence of cerebral infarction was 22% (67/278) in patients given nimodipine compared to 33% (92/276) in placebo-treated patients. In patients given nimodipine, final poor outcome occurred in 20% (55/278) versus 33% (71/276) in patients given placebo. The relative risks of cerebral infarction and poor outcome were significantly reduced by 34% and 40%, respectively. The conclusion was that nimodipine was well tolerated, reduced cerebral infarction, and improved outcome after SAH.

3. Discussion

Uncontrolled studies are open to criticism, especially when the effect of a new pharmacological agent is tested. The results of uncontrolled trials cannot be compared. In the case of nimodipine, uncontrolled single or multicentre studies showed spectacularly good results. It is impossible to determine if such favourable results were due to the judicious combination of expert neurosurgeons, early surgery, careful management and the tested drug or due to the effect of the drug itself. Nevertheless, all these uncontrolled studies suggest a favorable trend of nimodipine in decreasing the incidence of postoperative ischemic complications. In some studies, the rate of surgical complications were remarkably high, approaching 10 to 19%, greatly exceeding the rate of delayed ischemic deteriorations (Auer 1983, Auer *et al.* 1984, Hillman *et al.* 1988, Gilsbach and Harders 1989). In some studies, it was possible to calculate the number of early aneurysm operations done each year by each of the 4 to 6 neurosurgeons composing the team: surprisingly, the number was only 3 to 5 aneurysms per year by each neurosurgeon, if no prerogative existed for anyone in the team (Auer *et al.* 1986, Hillmann *et al.* 1988, Gilsbach and Harders 1989). All these studies, however, have contributed to the advancement of early aneurysmal surgery and the promotion of calcium antagonists in the prevention of postoperative ischemic deficit possibly due to vasospasm.

The results of controlled randomized trials are more convincing. Special attention must be drawn to the results of the British aneurysm nimodipine trial: oral nimodipine reduced by 34% the incidence of cerebral infarcts and by 40% the poor outcome after subarachnoid hemorrhage (Pickard *et al.* 1989). This is the best prospective placebo-controlled randomized multicentre study ever done to study the effects of nimodipine. It showed a reduction in the rate of severe cerebral ischemic deterioration after subarachnoid hemorrhage from 15–35% without nimodipine to 9–23% with the drug. However, in this trial, there is no evidence that nimodipine reduced the mortality due to cerebral ischemia: of the 39 patients given nimodipine who developed cerebral ischemia 17 (43.5%) died, compared to 25 (40.9%)

the 61 patients with cerebral ischemia who were given placebo. In the Canadian multicentre nimodipine study, it was found that poor-grade patients benefitted from oral nimodipine treatment. In these patients, nimodipine could reduce by 40% the risk of permanent ischemic deficit due to vasospasm alone or to vasospasm associated with another etiology (Petruk *et al.* 1988).

There is some discrepancy between the favourable clinical results and the less favourable results in a series of experimental SAH in primates. Nimodipine failed to reverse angiographic vasospasm and had no beneficial effect on the neurological symptoms in animals (Nosko *et al.* 1985). This lack of effect on vasospasm was also observed in some clinical studies, where nimodipine failed to increase the diameter of the intracranial spastic vessels seen as on follow-up angiography (Philippon *et al.* 1986, Petruk *et al.* 1988). Additionally, nimodipine did not increase significantly the CBF in patients treated with nimodipine (Messeter *et al.* 1987, Mee *et al.* 1988). In 24 patients receiving nimodipine postoperatively, Vinge *et al.* (1988) found that the serum thromboxane B2 concentration was not substantially different from patients who did not receive nimodipine, suggesting that nimodipine had no effect on platelet function in such patients. The mechanism of action of nimodipine on the cerebral circulation remains imperfectly understood, as its favourable effects are not angiographically measurable as might have been expected. Nimodipine may have a vasoactive effect on capillaries or provide neuronal protection against calcium disorders involved in ischemic brain damage (Brandt *et al.* 1988, Siesjö 1984). In a primate model of SAH, Dorsch *et al.* (1989) suggested that nimodipine may have a cellular protective effect against ionic changes due to ischemia, but does not affect significantly the CBF which was increased up to 16%. Presently, especially in the absence of any other treatment, some clinical arguments indicate a place of the calcium antagonist nimodipine in the medical management of patients admitted within 3 days after their aneurysmal SAH.

C. Nicardipine

Nicardipine hydrochloride, a water-soluble drug, is a 1,4-dihydropyridine derivative with cerebrovascular effects demonstrated in animals and human beings (Takenaka and Handa 1979, Yamamoto *et al.* 1983). Intravenous injection of 0.01 mg/kg of nicardipine increased cerebral blood flow by 17% with a minimal decrease in arterial blood pressure (Takenaka and Handa 1979). Nicardipine is essentially used as an antihypertensive drugs. Experimentally, it was demonstrated that nicardipine could significantly decrease the release of prostaglandins PGD2 and leucotrienes LTC4 and enhance the release of prostaglandin PGE2 (Rodriguez y Baena *et al.* 1989).

Effective serum concentrations were smaller after intravenous administration than after oral doses in both humans and animals, suggesting that the drug is readily eliminated by first-pass metabolism (Higuchi and Shiobara 1980). Nicardipine can be administered either orally or intravenously. Nicardipine for intravenous infusion is supplied in 10 ml ampules containing 10 mg of the drug. Tablets of 30 mg nicardipine are available, the recommended dosage being 90 to 120 mg per day. For intravenous infusion, it is better to add the drug to normal saline or to 5–10% glucose solution, the recommended dosage being 0.03 mg/kg/hour (approximately 2 mg/hour). If higher doses as up to 0.15 mg/kg/hour are infused, it is advisable to begin with a incremental dosage under control of the arterial blood pressure for six or eight hours at least (Flamm *et al.* 1988). No side effects other than hypotension have been reported (Flamm and Adams 1988). Treatment with intravenous nicardipine 0.03 mg/g/hour costs approximately 25 Francs per day (or 4 to 5 US Dollars).

A study of nicardipine dosage relationships was performed in 67 patients with recent aneurysmal subarachnoid hemorrhage admitted within 7 days after hemorrhage (Flamm *et al.* 1988). Patients were graded 1 to 5 on the author's personal scale similar to that of Hunt and Hess. Nicardipine was administered intravenously in a progressive fashion during the first four hours of the infusion, and thereafter at a constant dosage during 7 to 14 days. Antihypertensives, corticosteroïds, and antifibrinolytic drugs were also administered. Timing of surgery was optional. Two groups of patients were analysed according to the dosage of nicardipine: 34 patients in the group Dose Levels 1 to 6 received nicardipine infused at 0.8 to 7.8 mg/h (0.01 to 0.11 mg/kg/hour), and 33 patients were classified Dose Level 7 and received nicardipine infused at approximately 10.4 mg/hour (0.15 mg/kg/hour). Hypotension, equivalent to a blood pressure of 100 mmHg or less, was observed in 28.3% (19/67) of the patients and within the first 6 hours after initiation of the treatment in 15 of them. The overall morbidity and mortality were 7% (5/67) and 6% (4/67), respectively, and were comparable in both groups of patients. Delayed ischemic deficit affected 26,5% (9/34) of patients in the group Dose Levels 1 to 6, compared with 6.1% (2/33) of the patients given Dose Level 7. No patient died from an ischemic complication. In the follow-up angiogram performed on days 7 to 10, angiographic vasospasm was observed in 46% (31/67) of cases. This angiographic spasm was less frequent in patients treated with high doses: 24.2% (8/33) versus 67.6% (23/34). The conclusion was that nicardipine appears to prevent both angiographic vasospasm and cerebral ischemia after subarachnoid hemorrhage.

As part of the same study on intravenous nicardipine, 42 of 67 patients awaiting delayed surgery were treated with antifibrinolytics (aminocaproïc acid 1.5 g/hour) and intravenous nicardipine. Fifteen patients received nicardipine at Dose Levels 1 to 6 and 27 patients were treated with high Dose Level 7. Delayed ischemic deterioration with concomitant evidence of angiographic vasospasm occurred in 12% (5/47) of patients resulting on a cerebral infarction in only one case. Compared with the data from the Cooperative Aneurysm Study (34%) and the Dutch-British study (24%), this incidence of symptomatic vasospasm was notably low (Kassell *et al.* 1984, Vermeulen *et al.* 1984). Clinical outcome at three months showed 7.1% (3/42) morbidity and 7.1% (3/42) mortality. These favourable findings suggest that the incidence of vasospasm and cerebral infarction in patients treated with antifibrinolytic drugs can be reduced by the concomitant prescription of a calcium antagonist (Beck et al., 1988).

Conclusions on the efficiency of nicardipine in the prevention of cerebral vasospasm are impossible at present because large clinical controlled trials are still lacking. It would be interesting to know the results of the current placebo-controlled study still going on in North America. Whether it is relevant to further compare two calcium antagonists like nicardipine and nimodipine is doubtful. There is no theoretical evidence to suggest that nicardipine is more efficient and has fewer side effects than nimodipine.

D. Other Calcium Antagonists

1. Diltiazem

Diltiazem is a benzothiazepine derivative with an experimentally demonstrated vasoactive effect on cerebral arteries (Van Breeman *et al.* 1981, Bevan 1982). On the basis of a potent preventive effect on experimental chronic cerebral vasospasm in primates (Frazee *et al.* 1985, Frazee *et al.* 1988), the clinical use of diltiazem has been proposed in the prevention of vasospasm. Diltiazem was administered to 21 patients with subarachnoid hemorrhage (Saunders *et al.* 1986). Although the final results of this trial are not yet known, Saunders *et al.* (1986) reported hematologic complications due to diltiazem in 2 of their patients who developed an increased bleeding time greater than 15 minutes. The bleeding time normalized after diltiazem was discontinued. Most of the calcium antagonists inhibit platelet aggregation, diltiazem being here more potent than many other agents tested.

2. Flunarizine

The results of a prospective uncontrolled study in 72 patients with aneurysmal subarachnoid hemorrhage were favourable to early treatment with 0.7 mg/kg/hour intravenous flunarizine (Kim *et al.* 1989). The incidence of delayed ischemic deficits from vasospasm alone was 13.8% (10/72). Flunarizine was successfully administered at a dose of 10 mg four times daily to 37 consecutive patients who were operated on early from their ruptured intracranial aneurysm (Fujita et al. 1990). Only one patient developed permanent ischemic neurological deficit, and there were no side effects from flunarizine.

III. Other Drugs

A. Nizofenone

Nizofenone (Y 9179) is an imidazole derivative with protective properties against cerebral anoxia and ischemia due to its free radical scavenging action and its depressant action on the cerebral metabolic rate. Compared to barbiturates, nizofenone showed far less depressant action on the central nervous system and the cardiorespiratory system (Ochiai *et al.* 1982). The clinical effects of nizofenone in the prevention of cerebral ischemia after subarachnoid hemorrhage were tested in a placebo-controlled randomized multicentre study (Saïto *et al.* 1983). One hundred patients were included, 42 of them being assigned to nizofenone, 48 receiving placebo. Ten patients were secondarily excluded for severe non-detailed complications unrelated to vasospasm. Nizofenone 10 mg was administered three times per day intravenously with a slow infusion over 30 minutes. The decrease in the blood pressure was mild and transient, the drop averaging 9% and lasting 90 minutes. Outcome at one month was analyzed. There was no reduction in the incidence of symptomatic vasospasm. The morbidity plus mortality was 28.5% of patients given nizofenone, compared with 37.5% in the non-treated patients, a 24% relative reduction of risk. Nizofenone is not available for clinical or experimental use, except in Japan.

B. Reserpine + Kanamycin

The association of reserpine and kanamycin was proposed by Zervas and associates in the prevention of vasospasm and delayed ischemic deficit after subarachnoid hemmorhage. In experimental studies, Zervas *et al.* (1979) found that the combination of reserpine and kanamycin lowered the concentration of vasoactive amines in blood, preventing the development of vasospasm after cisternal injection of autologous blood. They also found that reserpine and kanamycin failed to reverse established vasospasm or to stop its progression. Both are capable of lowering blood serotonin concentration. Reserpine is a phosphodiesterase inhibitor and prevents storage of vasosactive amines like serotonin in patelets. Kanamycin is an intestinal antibiotic that interferes with the synthesis of pyridoxine necessary in the synthesis of serotonin. Reserpine and kanamycin administered after aneurysmal rupture cannot reduce the vasosactive properties of the initially extravated blood, and thus the incidence of preoperative vasospasm, but rather that occurring in the postoperative period due to peroperative hemorrhage in the area of operation.

A prospective placebo-controlled randomized study was carried out in 54 patients in clinical grade equivalent to Hunt and Hess grade 1 or 2 after their subarachnoid hemorrhage, 26 were assigned to treatment with subcutaneous reserpine 0.2 mg q.i.d. and oral kanamycin 400 mg t.i.d., 28 received placebo (Zervas *et al.* 1979). Preoperative clinical or angiographic vasospasm occurred in 12% (3/26) of the patients treated with the double drug therapy, and in 39% (11/28) of patients given placebo. The incidence of postoperative cerebral vasospasm was not statistically different, being 4.5% (1/22) in the treated group and 14.2% (4/28) in the other. Subsequently, Zervas *et al.* (1980) were not able to confirm the protective effect of this therapy, as in a new series of 28 patients treated the incidence of preoperative ischemic complications was 25%. Postoperative ischemic complications were, however, reduced to 4%.

The favourable results reported by Zervas *et al.* (1980) have never been confirmed by others. In a series of 10 patients who had serum serotonin level controlled below the normal range, Blumenkopf *et al.* (1980) found that the previous administration of reserpine and kanamycin or the reduction of serum serotonin level or plasma norepinephrine level were not associated with reduction in the incidence of ischemic deterioration. In a retrospective study, Knuckey and Stokes (1982) confirmed that kanamycin and reserpine did not protect against preoperative vasospasm, whereas they found that this treatment would reduce the incidence of postoperative vasospasm. Reserpine and kanamycin are no longer considered as drugs of potential interest in the prophylaxis of vasospasm in humans.

C. Anti-Thromboxane A2 Synthetase

It has been suggested that during the active phase of vasospasm following subarachnoid hemorrhage, an imbalance between synthesis of prostaglandin PG12 and thromboxane A2 may be an indirect cause of persistent vasospasm and of microthrombosis, leading to cerebral ischemic symptoms (Suzuki *et al.* 1981, Nosko *et al.* 1988). Excess of thromboxane A2 can reinforce vessel spasticity and lead to thrombosis of the spastic vessel or of perforating arteries. However, in an experimental primate model of subarachnoid hemorrhage, basal levels of prostacyclin and thromboxane A2 were measured in the cerebral vessels and the imbalance found in favour of thromboxane A2 not because of increase of its synthesis but on the contrary because of the relative lack of prostacyclin (Nosko *et al.* 1988).

For their properties of inhibition of the thromboxane A2 synthetase, the three following drugs have been administered to patients after aneurysmal subarachnoid hemorrhage:

— Trapidil: 5-methyl-7-diethylamino-s-triazolo-[1.5-a]-pyrimidine
— OKY 1581: sodium (E)-3-[4-(3-pyridylmethyl)-phenyl)]-2-propenoate
— OKY 046: sodium (E)-3-[4-(1-imidazolymethyl)-phenyl]-2-propenoate

Trapidil is a coronary vasodilator and an antagonist and selective synthesis inhibitor of thromboxane A2. Oral Trapidil 100 or 150 mg three times daily was given to 20 patients admitted in grade 1 to 4 of Hunt and Hess and operated on within 72 hours post-SAH (Suzuki *et al.* 1981). Angiographic vasospasm occurred in 9 cases (45%) but only 2 cases (10%) displayed mild ischemic symptoms due to vasospasm.

Tani *et al.* (1984) reported their clinical experience of OKY 1581 in 27 patients receiving the drug intravenously during the postoperative period after early surgery. These patients were compared to a group of 22 patients who did not receive the drug but were treated with hypertensive hypervolemia. No statistical difference was found in the incidence of postoperative angiographic vasospasm nor in the incidence of postoperative ischemic symptoms. The final outcome of the two groups of patients was similar. Low density areas on the postoperative CT scan associated with symptomatic vasospasm were, however, less frequent in the patients treated with the drug: 4 of 27 or 15% versus 10 of 22 or 45% of patients who did not receive the drug.

OKY 046 was administered intravenously in a prospective multicentre uncontrolled study (Suzuki *et al.* 1985). Eighty-two patients were treated and symptomatic vasospasm occurred in 33% (27/82) but with mild or transient neurological symptoms in 18 of them. Thereafter, the incidence of severe vasospasm was 10.9% (9/82). It was shown that OKY 046 decreased the blood of level thromboxane B2 the stable metabolite of thromboxane A2.

D. Heparin

Heparin accelerates the activity of antithrombin III, with the subsequent inhibition of factor X blocking the coagulation cascade. Heparin has paradoxically been proposed in the prophylaxis of symptomatic vasospasm because, experimentally, antithrombin III has been shown to relax basilar arteries precontracted by thrombin or plasmin, vasosactive agents believed to participate in the formation and maintenance of arterial vasospasm (White and Robertson 1987). Heparin may also prevent the proliferative angiopathy following subarachnoid hemorrhage. In experimental subarachnoid hemorrhage, heparin reduced the morphologic changes occurring in the arterial wall after SAH, by inhibition of the platelet-derived growth factor that stimulates the proliferation of fibroblasts and the growth or migration of smooth muscle cells of the vascular wall (Kapp *et al.* 1985). Heparin may reduce the adhesiveness of platelets on the injured arterial wall, limiting the size of platelet aggregates and the risk of micro-emboli. Heparin has no fibrinolytic activity, so it does not increase the risk of recurrent hemorrhage in aneurysmal subarachnoid hemorrhage once the fibrin clot is formed. However, the risk of transforming a recurrent minor leak into a dramatic major bleed with fatal intracerebral hemorrhage is likely to be higher in the presence of heparin.

In a retrospective clinical study, Kapp *et al.* (1987) reported favourable effects of heparin in the prevention of cerebral ischemic complications following gradual carotid ligation in 161 patients with ruptured intracranial aneurysms. One hundred and four patients received heparin and their results were compared with a group of 57 patients who were treated identically except for heparin. Ischemic neurological deficit occurred in 19.2% (20/104) of patients who received heparin, and 36.6% (22/57) of patients who did not receive the drug. Still more surprising was the lower incidence of rebleeding in the group of patients given heparin with a 9.6% incidence versus 26.1% in the non-treated group of patients. Although in this study the cerebral ischemia could have been due to hypoperfusion or emboli in relation with the carotid ligation, heparin may have prevented some ischemic deficits attributable to the presence of chronic vasospasm or proliferative angiopathy, or both. Even if heparin cannot be recommended routinely at present, it is possible that future clinical trials will confirme the role of new low molecular weight heparin in the prophylaxis of vasospasm (Chimowitz and Pessin 1987).

E. Dipyridamole

The role of a proliferative vasculopathy in the genesis of the postoperative delayed cerebral ischemic deficit is still debated. Excessive platelet adhesiveness may result from interaction of blood platelets and abnormal endothelial cells. Release of platelet micro-emboli could be an intravascular factor which combined with vasospasm leads to multifocal cerebral ischemia (Kassell *et al.* 1985, Bevan and Bevan 1988). Studying platelet adhesiveness in patients presenting with aneurysmal SAH, Laine *et al.* (1978) proposed prophylaxis with intravenous daily injection of 80 mg of dipyridamole or 300 mg/day of aspirin orally. In a prospective study the outcome of the 51 patients receiving the drug was reported to be substantially better compared to that of a large retrospective untreated group.

More recently, the effects of dipyridamole were tested in a clinical trial looking at the outcome of 677 patients presenting with SAH (Shaw *et al.* 1985). Patients were randomized on admission to receive placebo (341 patients) or dipyridamole (336 patients) in a standard oral dose of 100 mg/day or 10 mg/day intravenously. No significant differences were observed between the control and treatment groups.

F. *Ticlopidine*

Ticlopidine, a drug which modifies platelet aggregability, was administered to 101 of 139 patients admitted within 72 hours after subarachnoid hemorrhage (Kita *et al.* 1989). Thirty-eight patients were treated without ticlopidine. Fatal vasospasm was significantly less frequent in the treated group (6%) than in the untreated group (34%). In this controlled non-randomized prospective study, the results of the hemorrheological control suggested that patients who had fatal vasospasm presented coagulation abnormalities similar to disseminated intravasular coagulation.

Treatment of Symptomatic Vasospasm

Symptomatic vasospasm is a major complication occurring in the first two weeks after SAH and ascribed to arterial spasm leading to progressive delayed cerebral ischemia. This complication may be activated by various extrinsic or intrinsic factors, such as dehydration, hypovolemia, a surgical procedure, or even angiography. Clinically, the term "symptomatic vasospasm" may be ascribed to any delayed neurological deterioration occurring before or after aneurysm surgery, not related to the direct effect of the initial bleed, a recurrent hemorrhage or the development of hydrocephalus. Obviously, the term vasospasm is inappropriate to describe such a multifactorial etiology of cerebral ischemia occurring after subarachnoid hemorrhage, but as Symon (1980) stated "it is so ingrained in the literature and so neatly encompassing a variety of only partially defined problems, that we must perforce remain with it".

The clinical diagnosis of symptomatic vasospasm can rarely be made with certainty and often by exclusion. Thus, whatever the clinical findings suggesting symptomatic vasospasm, CT scan should be performed to rule out other sources of neurological deterioration. The following definition of preoperative and postoperative vasospasm may be proposed.

— Preoperative symptomatic vasospasm refers to an ischemic event occurring while the patient is awaiting surgery. The onset of this syndrome is delayed and progressive, occurring generally between day 5 and day 9 after SAH. This clinical event cannot be attributed to another complication such as rebleed or hydrocephalus. The neurological deficit is not always related to the site of the aneurysm. The cerebral ischemia is associated with the presence of focal or diffuse arterial vasospasm that may or may not be confirmed with transcranial doppler or on angiography (if performed).

— Postoperative symptomatic vasospasm refers to any neurological deficit occurring either after early or delayed operation for ruptured intracranial aneurysm. This neurological deterioration takes place in the absence of intraoperative complications or postoperative treatable events demonstrable on a CT scan such as extra-dural or intradural hemorrhagic collections, or hydrocephalus. This neurological deficit is delayed for some hours or even days after surgery and frequently is appropriate to the side of the operation. It is related to the development of a cerebral ischemia associated or not with an arterial vasospasm.

It is not clear that preoperative and postoperative ischemic neurological deficits have the same origin, but the same mechanism of action is generally admitted: reduction of CBF leading to cerebral ischemic complications. Regional CBF and oxygen utilization are significantly depressed in both hemispheres after subarachnoid hemorrhage (Grubb *et al.* 1977, Montgomery *et al.* 1981, Martin *et al.* 1984, Voldby *et al.* 1985, Hino *et al.* 1989, Yonas *et al.* 1989). Oxygen extraction is increased in both hemispheres signifying failure of the cerebral circulation to satisfy metabolic demand. Correlations between arterial pressure and the fluctuations in neurological deficit have been observed, suggesting that CBF and oxygen delivery can be improved by the elevation of the arterial blood pressure (Montgomery *et al.* 1981). The treatment of symptomatic vasospasm during the preoperative or the postoperative period is thus quite similar and directed towards improvement of cerebral perfusion pressure and/or reversal of the chronic arterial vasospasm.

To improve cerebral perfusion pressure it is necessary to control intracranial pressure and to increase the cardiac output using intravascular volume expansion with or without the addition of vasopressive drugs. Various vasoactive drugs against the persistent arterial vasospasm have been tried with limited effects (Wilkins 1986). To limit extension of the cerebral ischemia, to protect the patient from cerebral infarction and from intracranial hypertension due to extensive cerebral edema, various agents have been suggested. The usefulness of barbiturates, calcium antagonists or steroids, all drugs providing a metabolic neuronal protection, is controversial (Hashi and Tabaka 1980, Hashi *et al.* 1980, Kassell *et al.* 1980, Miyagi *et al.* 1984, Chyatte and Sundt 1984, Samson and Beyer 1980, Koos *et al.* 1985).

I. Hypervolemia and Hypertension

The most commonly successful treatment of delayed cerebral ischemia after SAH is intravascular volume expansion with or without elevation of the systolic blood pressure. Hypervolemia or hypertension have no chemical neuronal protective effect but improve the cerebral microcirculation through the following sequence: increase of intravascular volume – increase in cardiac output — improvement of CBF with concomitant improvement of the macrorheological and microrheological conditions of the intracerebral circulation. Hypervolemia or arterial hypertension should be applied with extreme caution before the aneurysm has been treated.

Clinical trials evaluating the beneficial effect of hypervolemia in the management of symptomatic vasospasm are lacking. Experimental and clinical findings have demonstrated the inability of intravascular volume expansion to increase CBF when autoregulation is preserved (Wood *et al.* 1982, Davis and Sundt 1980, Yamakami *et al.* 1987). Despite this, hypervolemic therapy has been widely recommended as the primary treatment of cerebral ischemia after SAH. The first results of hypervolemia were reported by Giannotta *et al.* (1977). Seventeen patients, who developed postoperative neurological deficits associated with angiographic vasospasm, were treated by arterial hypertension induced by hypervolemia and vasopressors if necessary. The results were favourable in 13 patients, unfavourable in 2 patients in whom a minor deficit persisted, and fatal in 2 patients. In 10 patients, intravascular volume expansion was enough to elevate the systolic blood pressure to an optimal level without the addition of vasopressive drug. Most of these were presumably included in the 13 patients who finally achieved a good outcome. In 10 patients who developed neurological deficit associated with angiographic vasospasm, hypervolemia alone gave excellent results in 9 (Tanabe *et al.* 1982). In these cases, infusion of albumin did not increase intracranial pressure.

Yamakami *et al.* (1987) measured CBF in 35 patients before and after a slight intravascular volume expansion achieved with 500 ml of 5% albumin. CBF significantly decreased after the infusion in all patients evaluated within the first two weeks after their SAH. During the third and fourth week post-SAH, CBF decreased only in patients with symptomatic vasospasm. In "normovolemic" patients, an increase in the cardiac output without significant elevation of the systolic blood pressure did not further increase CBF. These negative findings were corroborated by some experimental reports. Davis and Sundt (1980) stated that normal autoregulation could account for the lack of change in CBF when cardiac output is increased. In an experimental model of cerebral ischemia (multiple intracranial arterial ligation in dogs), intravascular volume expansion without hemodilution did not increase CBF either in the ischemic or the normal brain, even with a 42% cardiac output elevation (Wood *et al.* 1982). Experimentally, it was confirmed that the reduction of blood viscosity can account for the direct relationship between CBF and cardiac output (Wood *et al.* 1983, Wood *et al.* 1984).

It is likely that volume expansion achieved by intravenous infusion of plasma expanders rather than by erythrocyte transfusion leads to hemodilution with decrease in hemoglobin and hematocrit. Tanabe *et al.* (1982) reported that with albumin infusion, hematocrit fell from 40 to 27% within a few days and remained at a low level throughout the period of treatment. With cardiac output and pulmonary wedge pressure monitored via a Swan-Ganz catheter the loading volume can be adjusted and hematocrit maintained greater than 32% (Tanabe *et al.* 1988). The question of the optimal hematocrit in pathologic situations and especially after SAH is nicely discussed by Hino *et al.* (1989). Hemodilution was used with enthusiasm in the early treatment of cerebral ischemia (Grotta 1987, Heros and Korosue 1989). It is well known that a hematocrit of 33% provides the best tradeoff between blood viscosity and oxygen carrying capacity. The relationship between blood viscosity and cerebral blood flow has been experimentally assessed in cats (Muizelaar *et al.* 1986). A 20% reduction of hematocrit led to a 45% increase in CBF. Conversely, a 10% increase in hematocrit resulted in a 20% decrease in CBF. In normal situations, with a lower hematocrit, the oxygen carrying capacity is decreased. The increase in CBF is only a normal physiologic compensatory response to the reduction of hematocrit and blood viscosity (Muizelaar and Becker 1986). During hemodilution, the subsequent increase in CBF has not been shown to improve oxygen supply to the normal brain (Hino *et al.* 1989). Despite very attractive experimental results, the role of hemodilution in the management of patients with stroke is not yet defined (Italian Acute Stroke Study Group 1988, The Hemodilution in Stroke Study Group 1989). In the absence of any specific clinical trial, it is obviously premature to conclude that patients with symptomatic vasospasm after SAH will benefit from hemodilution.

Hypertension was first proposed by Denny-Brown (1951) in the treatment of cerebrovascular ischemic symptoms. Farhat and Schneider (1967) described four patients in whom metaraminol, a vasopressive drug, was successfully used. VanderArk and Pomerantz (1973) successfully treated a patient who postoperatively developed aphasia and motor deficit with metaraminol. The clinical symptoms cleared immediately although only partially after the blood pressure was elevated from 112/70 to 160/80 mmHg. In 1976, Kosnik *et al.* reported the results in seven patients who received arterial hypertension as a treatment of their postoperative neurological ischemic deficit. Volume expansion and norepinephrine were infused to elevate systolic blood pressure to 160 mgHg. All patients achieved a complete recovery except one who died. Koznik *et al.* (1976) emphasized the importance of starting the treatment as early as possible, claiming that 'to little and/or too late' may be worse than no treatment at all. Since then, there have been several other reports describing beneficial effect of hypertension and hypervolemia (Giannotta *et al.* 1977, Brown *et al.* 1978, Pritz *et al.* 1978, Ritchie *et al.* 1980, Tanabe *et al.* 1982, Solomon *et al.* 1984, Muizelaar and Becker 1986, Tanabe *et al.* 1988).

A. Hypervolemia

Intravascular volume expansion can be achieved by intravenous infusion of colloids. Crystalloïds are as effective as colloïds in restoring normal circulatory dynamics, but their administration may result in an increase of cerebral edema with subsequent intracranial hypertension (Heros and Korosue 1989). Low molecular weight dextran and human serum albumin or albumin derivatives are colloïds used routinely with a daily total perfused volume that may exceed 1500 ml. Hydroxyethyl starch is another colloïd solution with similar effects to low molecular weight-dextran, but less frequent allergic reactions or adverse renal effect. Human albumin has great advantages as it allows natural colloid osmotic pressure elevation with natural metabolic integration but 500 ml albumin 4–5% costs approximately 420–450 Francs, or 70–75 US Dollars. However, 500 ml infusion of a 4% albumin solution (20 g) contains 150 mmol sodium and 0.5 mmol potassium. The daily total weight of albumin that has been administered is reported to range between 0.5 g/kg/day to 2 g/kg/day (Tanabe *et al.* 1982, Yamakami *et al.* 1987). Due to the risk of viral disease transmission, the use of human serum, plasma, total blood or packed red blood cells should be abandoned. Optimal hypervolemia is achieved when the central venous pressure has increased from its 5–6 mmHg normal level to a 10 to 12 mmHg maximum level. Frequently, a moderate concomitant elevation of the systolic blood pressure occurs (plus 10 to 30 mmHg). Usually this elevation of the blood pressure is transient and reversed by the enhanced diuresis due to the increase in fluid intake.

Careful monitoring of pulse rate, central venous pressure, arterial blood pressure and continuous monitoring of ECG are strictly recommended (Pritz *et al.* 1978, Ritchie *et al.* 1980, Rosenwasser *et al.* 1983). In the elderly, or in patients with previous myocardial infarction or cardiac failure, hypervolemia cannot be safely applied in the absence of monitoring with a Swan-Ganz catheter. According to Pritz *et al.* (1978), such monitoring renders management of the hypervolemia safer since the permanent monitoring of pulmonary wedge pressure is more accurate than central venous pressure alone. The cardiac output and the cardiac index can also be assessed accurately both valuable parameters in the management of hypervolemia. Prophylactic administration of digoxine may also be used to

Table 4. *Structure of Endogenous and Synthetic Sympathomimetic Amines*

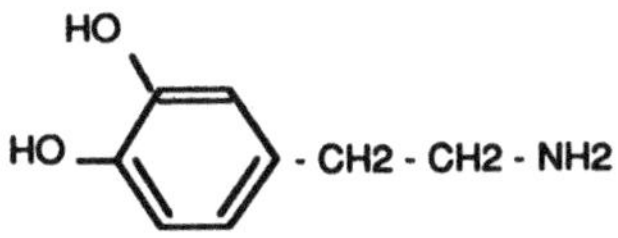

Dopamine

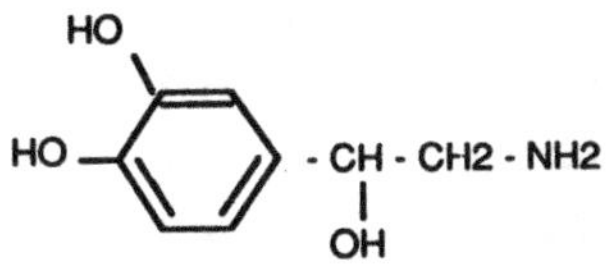

Norepinephrine

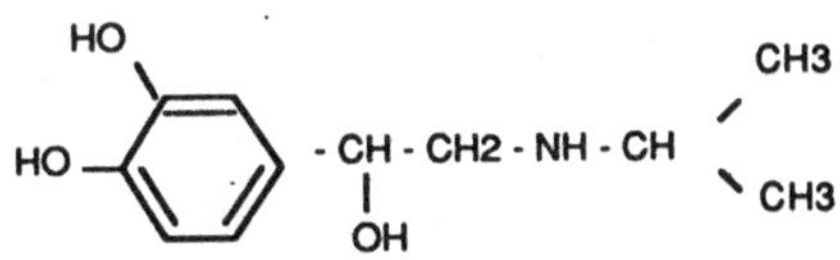

Isoproterenol

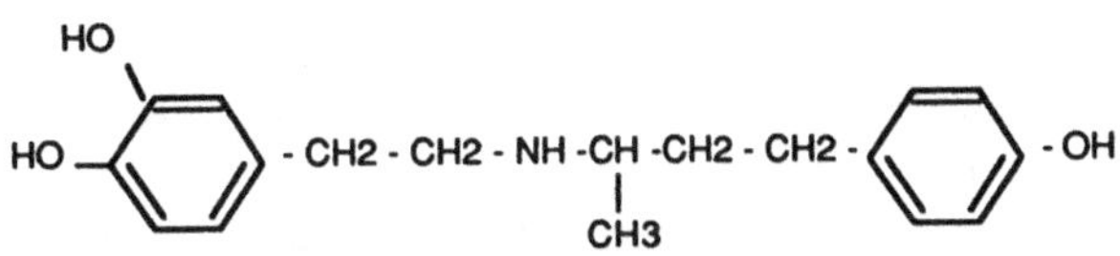

Dobutamide

improve cardiac function. Intravascular volume expansion can be successfully carried out even in hypertensive patients (Rosenwasser *et al.* 1983). Anti-hypertensive drugs as hydralazine, methyldopate, clonidine or even propanolol are preferable to vasodilators such as nifedipine, nicardipine or angiotensin converting-enzyme inhibitors. Diuretics should not be used.

Excessive volume expansion can lead to hemodynamic cardiac failure with subsequent pulmonary or renal dysfunction and intracranial hypertension. These adverse effects are reported by transient, being easily reversed by reduction of fluid intake, diuretics or digitalization (Giannotta *et al.* 1977, Kindt *et al.* 1980, Tanabe *et al.* 1982, Tanabe *et al.* 1988).

There is evidence that changes in intracranial presure occur during the first two weeks after SAH (Kaye and Brownbill 1981, Voldby *et al.* 1985, Takeuchi *et al.* 1989). Intracranial hypertension may well contribute to cerebral ischemia and clinical deterioration. Furthermore, as the blood-brain barrier is damaged, volume expansion may exacerbate ischemic cerebral edema. Continuous intracranial pressure monitoring should therefore always be carried out in patients presenting with severe neurological deterioration before commencing intravascular volume expansion. Intracranial pressure monitoring may be indicated also if there is a lack of response to treatment or if further deterioration occurs.

B. *Hypertensive Hypervolemia*

1. Vasopressive Drugs

The addition of vasopressive drugs to vascular volume expansion is often necessary to elevate the systolic blood pressure. Particularly indicated in case of acute left ventricular failure are Dopamine, Norepinephrine and drugs created by change in the structure of norepinephrine (epinephrine, isoproterenol, dobutamide). These elevate cardiac output and systolic blood pressure (see Table 4), and all augment myocardial contractility (positive inotropic effect) by direct stimulation of β1-adrenergic receptor sites in the myocardium. The clinical application of sympathomimetic drugs is limited by their positive chronotropic effects which cause tachycardia, induce arrhythmias, and increase myocardial oxygen consumption (Vasu *et al.* 1978). Furthermore, depending on their structure, catecholamines activate receptors other than cardiac β1-adrenergic receptors (see Table 5). The stimulation of alpha-adrenergic receptors causes peripheral vasoconstriction. The stimulation of β2-adrenergic receptors in the peripheral arterial system decreases peripheral resistance and thus decreases arterial pressure (Sonnenblick *et al.* 1979).

Norepinephrine is a potent alpha-adrenergic stimulator and a moderate β1-adrenergic stimulator and causes a substantial arterial pressure rise. This increase in peripheral vascular resistance can produce considerable hypertension from normal pressure levels. Norepinephrine is no longer available for clinical use in some countries.

Epinephrine is a alpha and β1-adrenergic stimulator and may be administered intravenously with doses varying on demand. Usually a response is obtained with doses between 0.001 mg/kg/min to 0.005 mg/kg/min. It has the same action as norepinephrine and is also no longer available for human use in all countries.

Dopamine, a precursor in the endogenous synthesis of norepinephrine, has a dose-dependent action on cardiac output and is administered intravenously. At a dose below 5 μg/kg/min it stimulates dopaminergic receptors causing mesenteric and renal vasodilatation with a subsequent increase in diuresis. Between 5 μg/kg/min to 20 μg/kg/min, dopamine stimulates β1 and β2-adrenergic receptors. In large doses (up to 20 μg/kg/min) dopamine may exert vasoconstrictive effects by stimulation of alpha-adrenergic receptors. Dopamine is known to have less prominent chronotropic effects than isoproterenol and less constrictive effects than norepinephrine (Sonnenblick *et al.* 1979). As dopaminergic effects are always present, intravenous administration of dopamine will always increase the urinary output.

Dobutamine is a synthetic catecholamine that directly increases myocardial contractility with less peripheral arterial effects or tachycardia than the other cited drugs (Sonnenblick *et al.* 1979). Its positive inotropic effect is similar to that observed with isoproterenol, a 56% increase in cardiac output for dobutamide and 63% for isoproterenol (Loeb *et al.* 1976). A 9% sinus rate increase has been observed with dopamine compared to the 17% increase in pulse rate observed with isoproterenol (Loeb *et al.* 1976). Dobutamide is administered intravenously at doses ranging from 2.5 μg/kg/min to 15 μg/kg/min.

2. Hypervolemia and Dopamine

Intravenous dopamine has been reported to be effective in the treatment of patients who developed an ischemic neurological deficit during the postoperative period and who did not respond to volume expansion (Giannotta *et al.* 1977, Brown *et al.* 1978, Haraguchi and Ebina 1982, Mendelow *et al.* 1986). A dose of dopamine as low as possible, mean levels reported from 9 to 46 μg/kg/min have been recommended. With a central venous pressure of 8 to 15 mmHg with volume expanders, dopamine infusion raised the arterial blood pressure up to 160–200 mgHg. The duration of treatment was 3 to 12 days.

Experimentally, dopamine was found to have a direct cerebral vasodilator effect which has been confirmed in patients (Battista *et al.* 1976, von Essen *et al.* 1980, Mendelow *et al.* 1986). After withdrawal of dopamine, CBF dropped from 34 ± 2 to 27 ± 2 ml/100 g/min on the ischemic hemisphere, and from 38 ± 3 to 32 ± 4 ml/100 g/min on the contralateral hemisphere. The differences between the mean cerebral blood flow values at highest and lowest doses of dopamine were statistically significant. During withdrawal of dopamine, 4 of the 8 patients treated deteriorated and treatment was resumed. All eight patients had a favourable outcome (Mendelow *et al.* 1986).

3. Hypertensive Hypervolemia

A series of 58 patients with preoperative or postoperative progressive severe neurological deficit associated with angiographic vasospasm were treated with hypervolemia and arterial hypertension (Kassell *et al.* 1982). Complete or partial resolution of the neurological deficit within one hour after the beginning of the treatment was observed in 81% (47/58). Permanent improvement occurred in 74% (43/58). Sixteen percent (9/58) remained unchanged and 10% (6/58) deteriorated during treatment. Interestingly, in

16 patients the deficit recurred when the blood pressure decreased transiently, and the clinical status was completely restored when the arterial pressure regained its previous level. In 16 patients with a recent subarachnoid hemorrhage and an unclipped aneurysm, the blood pressure was raised to more moderate levels, and three patients rebled as their systolic hypertension was elevated above 160 mmHg.

Hypervolemia plus hypertension needs continuous monitoring of central venous pressure and arterial pressure. Cardiac function should in addition be monitored with a Swan-Ganz catheter pulmonary arterial wedge pressure, cardiac output and the cardiac index then being continuously assessed. Usually with hypervolemic hypertension, the cardiac index rises up to 3 liters/min/sqm (Pritz *et al.* 1978). As in hypervolemic therapy, intracranial pressure monitoring is indicated when there is a severe neurological deficit and/or marked deterioration of the level of consciousness. The induction of hypervolemia and hypertension may lead to bradycardia and excessive diuresis. Atropine, 1 mg administered intramuscularly every 4 hours, may be necessary to control the vagal response (Kassell *et al.* 1982). Excessive diuresis should be compensated for by adequate fluid intake to maintain a positive fluid balance, and at times vasopressin or its synthetic derivatives are needed to keep the urine output down to 200 ml/hour (Kassell *et al.* 1982). Complications of hypervolemia with hypertension are related to overhydration with pulmonary edema, hemodilutional hyponatremia, cardiac failure or myocardial infarction, and thoracic or cardiovascular events in relation to the venous or Swan-Ganz catheters. Of course, patients are at risk to rebleeding if their aneurysm has not been treated.

4. Hypertension + Hypervolemia + Hemodilution

Patients operated on early can be treated at the first sign of clinical vasospasm with hypertensive hypervolemic hemodilution (H.H.H.). The results of this triple treatment has been reported in 41 patients admitted for ruptured intracranial aneurysm who presented preoperative or postoperative clinical deterioration attributed to vasospasm (Awad *et al.* 1987). Hemodilution was achieved by intravenous infusion of colloids. The hematocrit fell from 38.4 ± 3.3% on admission to 33.0 ± 1.9% during the course of treatment. Mean sodium concentration was not substantially modified by hemodilution. With hypervolemia from intravenous whole blood infusion, central venous pressure ranged between 10 to 12 mmHg. The systolic pressure was increased to 160–200 mmHg. In patients with an unclipped aneurysm, the systolic pressure never exceeded 120–150 mmHg. To reach the desired level of hypertension, it was necessary to add intravenous dopamine or other vasopressors in 39% (16/41) of the patients, under the control of a cardiologist. In hypertensive patients, the hypervolemia and the withdrawal of antihypertensive drugs were sufficient to obtain the desired level of hypertension. These results were considered encouraging as clinical improvement was noted in 60% of patients during the course of treatment. At the end of treatment, 47% (19/41) of patients were neurologically intact, 33% (14/41) had a minor neurological deficit, and 19% (8/41) had a bad outcome (1 major deficit, 7 deaths). Pulmonary edema was a complication in three cases who responded well to diuretics. No ischemic brain edema or hemorrhagic infarcts were reported.

Hypervolemia, hypervolemia plus dopamine, or hypertensive hypervolemia, and hypertensive hypervolemic hemodilution have the same rationale and are only progressive degrees of intensity of the same therapy. There is no evidence that clinical results obtained were substantially different between them. Usually, the more severe the clinical condition of the patient, the more aggressive was the treatment. This is particularly evident in the series where vasopressive drugs were added (Giannotta *et al.* 1977, Kassell *et al.* 1982, Awad *et al.* 1987). Either pre- or postoperatively, hypervolemia with or without hypertension is indicated as the first line of treatment in the presence of clinical deterioration attributable to cerebral ischemia. The following are recommended:

— Hypervolemia should be used first. When available, colloïds are preferred to any other volume expanders.

— Monitoring of central venous pressure is necessary. Hypervolemia is achieved when the central venous pressure stands between 6 and 12 mmHg, with no change in the systolic blood pressure. The hematocrit should not be below 31–33%.

— Hypertensive therapy is indicated in the absence of substantial clinical neurological improvement within four hours after hypervolemia has been achieved. If vasopressors are needed, dopamine is easier to manage, but need careful fluid balance control.

— The association of calcium antagonists with hypertensive hypervolemic therapy remains to be further evaluated as the blood-brain barrier may be modified with loss of autoregulation, and experimental evidence suggests the possible extension of vasogenic edema (Höllerhage *et al.* 1988).

II. Vasoactive Drugs

A. Isoproterenol + Lidocaïne

Sundt reported his experience with isoproterenol and lidocaïne in the treatment of preoperative cerebral vasospasm in 1973. In 14 patients with ischemic neurological deficit, the initial response to treatment was an arrest of progressive deterioration with definite improvement in 12 patients and no effect in 2 patients who died. The rationale of this treatment expected an intracranial arterial vasodilatation with isoproterenol, a β-adrenergic drug that dilates peripheral arterioles, and increases myocardial contractility with subsequent increase of the cardiac output, while Lidocaïne was proposed as an addition to limit the positive chronotropic effect of isoproterenol (Sundt *et al.* 1973). This favourable experience was confirmed later in 30 patients, 21 with excellent or good outcome, 7 poor final results, and 2 deaths (Sundt 1975).

B. Isoproterenol + Aminophylline

In 1976, Flamm found the combination of isoproterenol and aminophylline to be very active in the treatment of experimental chronic vasospasm. Isoproterenol was supposed to stimulate adenyl-cyclase while aminophylline simultaneously inhibited phosphodiesterases. Relaxation of the smooth muscle cell was then favoured, as the cyclic monophosphates controlled the intracellular influx of calcium which is essential for maintaining actin-myosin coupling (Flamm and Ransohoff 1976). Furthermore, it was postulated that this combined therapy might play a favourable role on the balance between prostacyclin and thromboxane A2 (Flamm 1980). With the combination of intravenous 125 μg/hour isoproterenol and 125 mg/hour aminophylline, improvement in neurological status of patients presenting with preoperative symptomatic vasospasm was observed in about 60% of the cases (Flamm and Ransohoff 1976, Fleischer *et al.* 1977, Flamm 1980, Fleischer and Tindall 1980, George *et al.* 1984). There was a rapid response in patients who tolerated this treatment. If the pulse rate increased over 140 per minute, the rate of infusion was reduced without addition of any other drug. The duration of this treatment varied from 5 days to 2 weeks. Patients severely affected, however, had a 40% mortality rate. A series of 32 patients presenting with preoperative angiographic vasospasm with or without clinical signs or clinical signs with decreased CBF was treated with the association of isoproterenol + aminophylline (George *et al.* 1984). The mortality was 37.5% and morbidity was 22.5%. This double-drug therapy was recommended with a monitoring of the central venous pressure and with volume expansion with albumin or plasminate before starting the treatment. Aminophylline and isoproterenol were administered with an infusion pump at a rate of 1.5 mg/kg/hour for aminophylline and 1.5 μg/kg/hour for isoproterenol. The medication was discontinued after three days if no improvement occurred and was continued for up to 14 days in case of favourable response.

This treatment was not well tolerated by some patients who developped tachycardia and cardiac arrythmias. Isoproterenol has a well-known positive chronotropic effect (Sonnenblick *et al.* 1979). This treatment is thus not indicated in patients with preexisting cardiac dysfunction, as the drug can cause arrythmias and premature atrial or ventricular complexes. The hemodynamic effect of isoproterenol is probably due more to its inotropic cardiac effect than to its β-adrenergic effect on the cerebral arteries. Other cardiac-active catecholamines are preferred to isoproterenol for their comparable inotropic because of their less pronounced chronotropic effect (Loeb *et al.* 1976).

Aminophyline is the water-soluble salt of theophylline. There is a strong relationship between toxicity and plasma concentration. The rate of drug metabolism can be modified by the clinical status of the patient, for example, hepatic cirrhosis increases by four the half-life time which is normally around 8 hours. Adverse reactions or toxic effects are associated with plasma theophylline concentration above 15 to 20 μg/ml. Tachycardia is the most common adverse side effect, preceding more serious adverse reactions such as cardiac arrythmias or seizures. Permanent brain damage or even death have been reported (Bailey *et al.* 1981). It is thus advisable to start the treatment with a standard loading dose of 8.0 mg/kg infused intravenously within thirty minutes to achieve a serum concentration between 10 and 20 μg/ml, and then adjust the infusion rate based on serial plasma theophylline assays (Bailey *et al.* 1981).

There are experimental arguments against this combined treatment. First, it was confirmed that intracarotid injection of aminophylline in man acts as a cerebral vasoconstrictor, reducing CBF even after infusion of small amounts (Gottstein and Paulson 1972). Secondly, isoproterenol has a low ability to cross the blood-brain barrier in man with a 3.8% extraction in a single passage because of its hydrosolubility (Olesen *et al.* 1978). Thirdly, intracarotid isoproterenol caused a significant reduction of CBF before the correction of a concomitant decrease in arterial pCO2 (Olesen *et al.* 1978). Additionally, experimental delayed cerebral vasospasm in dogs failed to be reversed by aminophylline treatment (Varsos *et al.* 1983).

C. Aminophylline + Nitroprusside + Dopamine

The addition of aminophylline to sodium nitroprusside and dopamine might be expected to have a synergistic favourable effect. Levy *et al.* (1982) reported the result of a combination of these three drugs administered intravenously in 5 patients presenting with evident delayed cerebral ischemia after aneurysmal SAH, who did not respond prior to volume expansion therapy. Aminophylline was started with a loading dose of 500 mg, and then was administered at 1 mg/kg/hour. Dopamine was slowly administered beginning at a dose of 1 to 5 μg/kg/min, until the blood pressure reached an optimal level. The dopamine infusion never exceeded 15 μg/kg/min. The nitroprusside dosage was variable but was never above 4 μg/kg/min. Practically, the doses varied from patient to patient. Theophylline and thyocyanate levels were monitored throughout. All patients responded favourably within 6 hours after the triple-drug therapy started. The improvement was sustained, and the treatment was stopped after two days without any weaning problems. This treatment combines cerebral vasodilation and increased cardiac output without causing excessive arterial hypertension (in four patients the ruptured aneurysm had not been secured). The results were encouraging, as all these patients who did not respond to hypervolemia showed a rapid and sustained response to this triple-drug therapy.

D. Nimodipine

Intravenous nimodipine has been proposed as an effective treatment of pre- or postoperative cerebral ischemia associated with vasospasm. In an uncontrolled prospective multicentre study, nimodipine was administered in 109 patients (Koos *et al.* 1985). Nimodipine was administered intravenously (24–48 mg/day) for 7 to 10 days and then orally (240 mg/day). Eighteen patients were later excluded. The results were reported in 91 patients. 60 patients presented preoperative clinical signs of cerebral ischemia, and 31 patients did so postoperatively. While 66% of the patients were admitted in Hunt and Hess grade 1 or 2, 84% of the patients were in grade 3 to 5 at the onset of the treatment. At the end of the treatment, a favourable outcome occurred in 65% (59/91) of the patients, while 22% (20/91) of the patients did not improve and 13% (12/91) died. No adverse effects occurred. Information about associated treatment or medical or surgical complications was reported.

In a French randomized placebo controlled multicentre prospective study (Jan *et al.* 1988), a trend towards better results was found in a series of patients treated with 0.03 mg/kg/hour of nimodipine intravenously. Patients were eligible for the study when they presented either with a neurological deterioration attributable to cerebral vasospasm and/or marked angiographically confirmed vasospasm. Among 188 eligible patients treated, 61 patients were later excluded for protocol violation. 73 patients received nimodipine and 54 patients received placebo. Mortality or morbidity were not statistically different between treated and non-treated patients in the total group of 188 patients. However, among the 127 validated cases, a separate analysis of the 77 patients presenting delayed ischemic deficit only due to vasospasm showed a significant statistical difference in morbidity and/or mortality. The outcome was less unfavourable in patients receiving nimodipine (8/42 or 19%) than in untreated patients (17/35 or

49%). The risk of morbidity or mortality was reduced by 61% in the treated group (49%–19% / 49% = 61%). In this study there is some confusion between patients included with symptoms due to vasospasm associated with angiographic signs and those included only with angiographic signs. Because of its rate of exclusions, the lack of information about the time of operation and the entrance date, and some statistical aspects, this study is open to criticism (Dorsch and Little 1989).

Intra-arterial nimodipine has been tried as a starting treatment of vasospasm during or after the angiography procedure (Grotenhuis *et al.* 1984, and Boker *et al.* 1985). In a series of 7 patients, Grotenhuis *et al.* (1984) concluded that intracarotid or intravertebral injection of nimodipine was not effective after vasospasm occurred, the immediate angiographic appearance remaining unchanged. Intravenous nimodipine was continued after the slow intra-arterial bolus, and the vasospasm was then judged less severe in some patients who had a third angiogram a week later. Boker *et al.* (1985) gave intra-arterial nimodipine to three patients in a dose of 0.2 mg/hour for 90 minutes. The intra-arterial infusion was not followed by clinical improvement, but in two cases the immediate repeat angiography revealed some resolution of the intracranial arterial narrowing. Subsequent standard intravenous treatment of nimodipine regime was used and the patients were successfully operated on with a good outcome in all three cases.

Unfortunately, there is no strong evidence that nimodipine can reverse signs and symptoms of pre- or postoperative cerebral ischemia from vasospasm with more efficacy than other forms of treatment. Increase in the dosage of intravenous nimodipine has not be reported to be more effective (Hillmann *et al.* 1988, Seiler *et al.* 1988).

III. Naloxone

In 1981, Baskin and Hosobuschi reported spectacular clinical improvement of ischemic deficits in three patients within four minutes after intravenous injection of 0.4 mg naloxone. This effect lasted for 20 minutes and then promptly disappeared. As the deficit in one of their patients was exacerbated by morphine, it was suggested that the use of analgesic agents acting on opiate receptors (even the codeïne so commonly used) in the treatment of headache after SAH should be avoided.

The role of naloxone, an opiate antagonist, in the management of patients with cerebral ischemia remains controversial. The confusion may have resulted from differences in methodology or treatment dose, or from an excessive simplification of the complex mechanism of action of opiate antagonists (Faden 1984). The role of naloxone on cerebral ischemia remains unknown, and a vasoactive role has been also attributed to the alkylparabens used as the vehicle in the parenteral preparation of naloxone hydrochloride (Bell *et al.* 1985). Furthermore, even if the clinical phenomenon of cerebral ischemia can be reversed, it is not clear that this was an effect of naloxone on the pathological process itself.

Naloxone must be given parenterally. After a single bolus naloxone concentration in the brain and in the blood falls rapidly. Thus, a constant infusion is necessary if a sustained action is to be achieved. Side effects of large doses of naloxone have been determined in a dose-response study confirming that large doses of naloxone did not produce major cardiovascular complications (Adams *et al.* 1986).

No significant beneficial effect of 0.4 mg of naloxone was evident later from a series of 21 patients with mild neurological deficits secondary to aneurysmal SAH (Bell *et al.* 1985), but a higher dose of 2.0 mg favourably (although marginally) changed the neurological condition in 5 patients, perhaps justifying further study in humans. The absence of clinical effects with low doses of naloxone do not justify any reserve in the use of codeïne or small doses of opiate agents for post-SAH headache (Bell *et al.* 1985). Naloxone may differentiate between reversible versus irreversible cerebral ischemia when injected as an intravenous bolus of 0.8 mg in patients with stroke (Estañol *et al.* 1985).

IV. Barbiturates

High dose barbiturate therapy in the treatment of neurological conditions associated with cerebral ischemia and/or intracranial hypertension has given rise to much controvery, as there is still no definitive proof that this therapy is effective in humans. Experimentally favourable effects of barbiturates on cerebral ischemia or intracranial hypertension have been demonstrated. This "brain protection" is supposed to result from the combined effects of a decrease in cerebral metabolic rate, a reduction of brain swelling and intracranial hypertension, an increase in the local tissue perfusion pressure, and membrane stabilization (Kassell *et al.* 1980). Furthermore, experimental in vitro relaxation of arterial tone previously increased by noradrenalin or potassium chloride or 5 hydroxytryptamine has been shown when pentobarbital was added in the circumstances of an organ bath (Marin *et al.* 1981).

When a progressive neurological deficit from vasospasm secondary to subarachnoid hemorrhage is refractory to any other aggressive treatment, this treatment has been proposed without any convincing clinical results (Hashi and Tabaka 1980, Kassell *et al.* 1980, Samson and Beyer 1980, Miyagi *et al.* 1984). All available clinical data pertains to less than 50 patients. The mortality neared 50%, but it is not obvious that this was the result of lack of effect or the consequence of management complications. Until further evidence of utility high dose barbiturate therapy should be limited to patients with severe diffuse cerebral ischemia from vasospasm unresponsive to any other treatment, and must, even then, be regarded as highly speculative.

V. Steroids

A. Hydrocortisone in Large Doses

In cats, after intravenous injection of large doses of hydrocortisone, a marked decrease in the spontaneous electrical activity recorded from the renal sympathetic nerve was documented (Hashi *et al.* 1980). Furthermore, suppression of vasoconstrictor tone in the cerebral vasculature was documented in dogs after 100 mg/kg intravenous injection of hydrocortisone, resulting in significant angiographic dilation. However, this intravenous injection was followed by bradycardia and a 50% drop of the arterial blood pressure. In the treatment of cerebral vasospasm, hydrocortisone in large doses was regarded as causing cerebral arterial dilatation with the prevention of cerebral edema.

This treatment was given to ten patients operated on within four days after the rupture of their intracranial aneurysm (Hashi *et al.* 1980). All patients developed 2 to 9 days later a deterioration of their consciousness with or without focal signs. The hydrocortisone intravenous dose was 100 mg/kg injected within 5 to 10 minutes twice daily, and the expected fall in arterial blood pressure was compensated by infusion of dopamine. Five patients improved clinically within 4 hours after the initial dose of hydrocortisone. The final outcome was excellent in 5 patients, poor in one case, and 4 patients died. Glycosuria exceeding 300 mg/dl was noted in 3 patients and required insulin injection. Gastro-intestinal hemorrhage occurred in one patient.

B. Dexamethasone, Betamethasone, Methylprednisolone

Dexamethasone, betamethasone or methylprednisolone are often used as part of the medical management of patients in poor condition after their aneurysmal SAH. It is surprising to find how frequently steroids are routinely prescribed to all patients admitted, as if it was a standard part of the medical management of aneurysmal SAH (Pritz *et al.* 1978, Giannotta *et al.* 1979, Zervas et al 1979, Kassell *et al.* 1980, Rosenwasser *et al.* 1983, Flamm *et al.* 1988, Öhman and Heiskanen 1988, Seiler *et al.* 1988, Gilsbach and Harders 1989). The usual dose administered is intravenous or intramuscular injection of 4 mg to 6 mg every 6 hours of dexamethasone or betamethasone, or 20 to 40 mg every 6 hours for prednisolone. To our knowledge, there has never been any validation of steroid therapy in such dosage in cases of SAH.

Various mechanisms of action have been proposed for possible steroid effect including free radical scavenging, lyzozyme membrane stabilization, mitochondrial stabilization, improved recovery of the energy metabolism. Only experimental data has ever suggested that steroids may prevent chronic cerebral vasospasm (Chyatte *et al.* 1983, Chyatte and Sundt 1984). The postulate was that chronic cerebral vasospasm may be linked to an inflammatory process following SAH. In dogs with SAH, large doses of methylprednisolone, dexamethasone or ibuprofen have been tested. A protective effect against cerebral vasospasm was confirmed with high doses of methylprednisolone (30 mg/kg every 8 hours), lower doses of methylprednisolone or usual doses of dexamethasone (0.1 mg/kg) were less effective although better than no treatment at all (Chyatte and Sundt 1984).

Twenty one patients with recent aneurysmal SAH considered to be at a high risk of delayed cerebral ischemia were treated with large doses of methylprednisolone (Chyatte *et al.* 1987). The intravenous treatment was 30 mg/kg every 6 hours, with a progessive withdrawal of the drug after 3 days. A group of 21 patients admitted at the same time served as controls. Delayed cerebral ischemia occurred in 5 of 21 treated patients, and in 9 of 21 non-treated patients. The mortality was higher in the control group than in the group of treated patients (28% versus 14%). Although the final outcome seemed substantially better in the group of treated patients, the results did not reach statistical significance. In this study, patients receiving high dose steroids developed neurological symptoms of cerebral ischemia later than expected, and it was suggested that the treatment could have delayed pathological events related to the inflammatory response. The toxic effects of prolonged high dose steroid treatment were briefly discussed. While steroids may have potential effect in minimizing ischemic cerebral damage, there is currently no proof of an effect on symptomatic vasospasm. Specific clinical trials are still lacking. In a placebo controlled randomized study, it has been shown the absence of any demonstrable beneficial effect of dexamethasone one the mortality and morbidity of spontaneous intracerebral hemorrhage and the presence of significant harmful effect, i.e., infections and exacerbation of diabetes has been shown (Poungvarin *et al.* 1987). This study suggested that after aneurysmal rupture with intracerebral hemorrhage, any effect of steroid treatment is questionable.

Conclusions

1. In the early management of aneurysmal SAH, there is a clear evidence that a number of manoeuvres can reduce the incidence of the major complications occurring within the first two weeks. and thereby can affect the final outcome of the patients. From the clinical studies reported, there is convincing evidence in favour of a positive preventive or curative effect of

the careful correction or overcorrection of the volemia. There is still a persistent doubt about the real efficacy of prevention provided by some of the drugs that are available.

2. Various pharmacological agents have been studied in patients, but only few of them have been really tested comparatively on a scientific basis. Double-blind controlled trials have been considered the best way to validate the clinical usefulness of a new drug. Controlled clinical trials are not always possible, however, because they require large financial and scientific supports, not always proportionate to the possible market value of the drug in terms of cost/effectiveness.

3. In the management of aneurysmal SAH, it is disappointing to find that after so many years clinical results have not been dramatically improved. This contrasts strongly with extraordinary efforts of experimental research. Experimental findings lead to a better understanding of the phenomena of cerebral arterial vasospasm; they emphasize for example the role of the endothelium in the reactivity of the cerebral arteries after SAH. It is now time for experimental findings to give rise to original clinical investigations.

References

1. Abenerthy DR, Schwartz JB (1988) Pharmacokinetics of calcium antagonists under development. Clin Pharmacokinet 15: 1–14
2. Adams HP (1987) Antifibrinolytics in aneurysmal subarachnoid hemorrhage. Do they have a role? Maybe. Arch Neurol 44: 114–115
3. Adams HP Jr, Nibbelink DW, Torner JC *et al* (1981) Antifibrinolytic therapy in patients with aneurysmal subarachnoid hemorrhage. A report of the cooperative aneurysm study. Arch Neurol 38: 25–29
4. Adams, HP, Olinger CP, Barsan WG *et al* (1986) A dose-escalation study of large doses of naloxone for treatment of patients with acute cerebral ischemia. Stroke 17: 404–409
5. Allen GS, Ahn HS, Preziosi TJ *et al* (1983). Cerebral arterial spasm: a controlled trial of nimodipine in patients with subarachnoid hemorrhage. N Engl J Med 308: 619–624
6. Alvarez Garijo JA, Vilches JJ, Aznar JA (1980) Preoperative treatment of ruptured intracranial aneurysms with tranexamic acid and monitoring of fibrinolytic activity. J Neurosurg 52: 453–455
7. Ameen AA, Illingworth R (1981) Antifibrinolytic treatment in the pre-operative management of subarachnoid hemorrhage caused by ruptured intracranial aneurysm. J Neurol Neurosurg Psychiatry 44: 220–226
8. Andreoli A, di Pasquale G, Pinelli G *et al* (1987) Subarachnoid hemorrhage: frequency and severity of cardiac arrhythmias. A survey of 70 cases studied in the acute phase. Stroke 18: 558–564
9. Aoyagi N, Hayakawa I (1984) Analysis of 223 ruptured intracranial aneurysms with special reference to rerupture. Surg Neurol 21: 455–452

10. Arieff AI, Ilach F, Massry SG (1976) Neurological manifestations and morbidity of hyponatremia: correlation with brain water and electrolytes. Medicine 55: 121–129
11. Auer LM (1983) Acute surgery of cerebral aneurysms and prevention of symptomatic vasospasm. Acta Neurochir (Wien) 69: 273–281
12. Auer LM (1984) Acute operation and preventive nimodipine improve outcome in patients with ruptured cerebral aneurysms. Neurosurgery 15: 57–66
13. Auer LM, Brandt L, Ebeling U *et al* (1986) Nimodipine and early aneurysm operation for good conditions SAH patients. Acta Neurochir (Wien) 82: 7–13
14. Awad IA, Carter LP, Spetzler RF *et al* (1987) Clinical vasospasm after subarachnoid hemorrhage: response to hypervolemic hemodilution and arterial hypertension. Stroke 18: 365–372
15. Bailey RT, Young B, Rapp RP *et al* (1981) Theophylline toxicity after the use of aminophylline in the treatment of cerebral vasospasm. Neurosurgery 9: 722–724
16. Baskin DS, Hosobuschi Y (1981) Naloxone reversal of ischemic neurological deficits in man. Lancet 2: 272–275
17. Battista AF, Flamm ES, Golstein M *et al* (1976) Effect of dopamine-beta-hydroxylase inhibition on cerebral vasospasm in the cat. J Neurosurg 44: 168–172
18. Beck W, Adams HP, Flamm ES *et al* (1988) Combination of aminoproïc acid and nicardipine in the treatment of aneurysmal subarachnoid hemorrhage. Stroke 19: 63–67
19. Bell BA, Miller JD, Neto NGF *et al* (1985) Effect of naloxone on deficits after aneurysmal subarachnoid hemorrhage. Neurosurgery 16: 498–501
20. Bevan JA (1982) Selective action of diltiazem on cerebral vascular smooth muscle in the rabbit: antagonism on extrinsic but not intrinsic maintained tone. Am J Cardiol 49: 519–524
21. Bevan JA, Bevan RD (1988) Arterial wall changes in chronic cerebrovasospasm: in vitro and in vivo pharmacological evidence. Ann Rev Pharmacol Toxicol 28: 311–329
22. Blumenkopf B, Wilkins RH, Feldmann JM (1980) Cerebral vasospasm and delayed neurological deficit after aneurysm rupture despite administration of reserpine and kanamycin. In: Wilkins RH (ed) Cerebral arterial spasm. Williams & Wilkins, Baltimore/London, pp 518–524
23. Böker DK, Solymosi L, Wassmann H (1985) Immediate postangiographic intraarterial treatment of cerebral vasospasm after subarachnoid hemorrhage with nimodipine. Neurochirurgia (Stuttg) 28: 118–120
24. Brandt L, Andersson KE, Ljunggren B *et al* (1988) Cerebrovascular and cerebral effects of nimodipine — an update. In: Reulen HJ, Philippon J (eds) Prevention and treatment of delayed ischaemic dysfunction in patients with subarachnoid hemorrhage. Acta Neurochir (Wien) [Suppl] 45. Springer, Wien New York, pp 11–20
25. Brouwers PJAM, Wijdicks EFM, Hasan D *et al* (1989) Serial electrocardiographic recording in aneurysmal subarachnoid hemorrhage. Stroke 20: 1162–1167

26. Brown FD, Hanlon K, Mullan S (1978) Treatment of aneurysmal hemiplegia with dopamine and mannitol. J Neurosurg 49: 525–529
27. Brown JA, Wollmann RL, Mullan S (1982) Myopathy induced by e-aminocaproïc acid. J Neurosurg 57: 130–134
28. Burchiel KJ, Hoffman JM, Bakay RAE (1984) Quantitative determination of plasma fibrinolytic activity in patients with ruptured intracranial aneurysms who are receiving e-aminocaproïc acid: relationship of possible complications of therapy to the degree of fibrinolytic activity. Neurosurgery 14: 57–63
29. Chimowitz MI, Pessin MS (1987) Is there a role for heparin in the management of complications of subarachnoid hemorrhage? Stroke 18: 1169–1172
30. Chyatte D, Fode NC, Nicholas DA *et al* (1987) Preliminary report: effects of high dose methylprednisolone on delayed cerebral ischemia in patients at high risk for vasospasm after subarachnoid hemorrhage. Neurosurgery 21: 157–160
31. Chyatte D, Rusch N, Sundt TM (1983) Prevention of chronic experimental vasospasm with ibuprofen and high dose methylprednisolone. J Neurosurg 59: 925–932
32. Chyatte D, Sundt TM (1984) Response of chronic experimental cerebral vasospasm to methylprenisolone and dexamethasone. J Neurosurg 60: 923–926
33. Cort JH (1954) Cerebral salt wasting. Lancet 1: 752–754
34. Crompton MR (1963) Hypothalamic lesions following the rupture of cerebral berry aneurysms. Brain 86: 301–314
35. Cruickshank JM, Neil-Dwyer G, Brice J (1974) Electrocardiographic changes and their prognostic significance in subarachnoid hemorrhage. J Neurol Neurosurg Psychiatry 37: 755–759
36. Cruickshank JM, Neil-Dwyer G, Stott AW (1975) Possible role of oral propanolol upon the ECG changes occurring in subarachnoid hemorrhage. Cardiovasc Res 9: 236–245
37. Davis DH, Sundt TM (1980) Relationship of cerebral blood flow to cardiac output, mean arterial blood pressure, blood volume, and alpha and beta blockade in cats. J Neurosurg 52: 745–754
38. Decaux G, Unger J, Brimioulle S *et al* (1982) Hyponatremia in the syndrome of inappropriate secretion of antidiuretic hormone. Rapid correction with urea, sodium chloride, and water restriction therapy. JAMA 247: 471–474
39. Denny-Brown D (1951) The treatment of recurrent cerebrovascular symptoms and the question of "vasospasm". Med Clin North Am 35: 1457–1474
40. Diringer M, Ladenson PW, Stern BJ *et al* (1988) Plasma atrial natriuretic factor and subarachnoid hemorrhage. Stroke 19: 1119–1124
41. Diringer M, Ladenson PW, Borel C (1989) Sodium and water regulation in a patient with cerebral salt wasting. Arch Neurol 46: 928–930
42. Doczi T, Bende J, Huska E *et al* (1981) Syndrome of inappropriate secretion of antidiuretic hormone after subarachnoid hemorrhage. Neurosurgery 9: 394–397
43. Doczi T, Joo F, Vecsernyés M *et al* (1988) Increased concentration of atrial natriuretic factor in the cerebrospinal fluid in patients with aneurysmal sub-

arachnoid hemorrhage and raised intracranial pressure. Neurosurgery 23: 16–19

44. Dorsch NWC, Branston NM, Harris RJ *et al* (1989) An experimental study of the effect of Nimodipine in primate subarachnoid hemorrhage. Acta Neurochir (Wien) 99: 65–75
45. Dorsch NWC, Little JM (1989) Reference: Nimodipine in cerebral vasospasm. Neurosurgery 24: 959–960
46. Doshi R, Neil-Dwyer G (1980) A clinicopathological study of patients following subarachnoid hemorrhage. J Neurosurg 52: 295–301
47. Estañol B, Aguilar F, Corona T (1985) Diagnosis of reversible versus irreversible cerebral ischemia by the intravenous administration of naloxone. Stroke 16: 1006–1009
48. Estañol BV, Badui Dergal E, Cesarman E *et al* (1979) Cardiac arrhythmias associated with subarachnoid hemorrhage: prospective study. Neurosurgery 5: 675–680
49. Estañol BV, Loyo MV, Mateos JH *et al* (1977) Cardiac arrhythmias in experimental subarachnoid hemorrhage. Stroke 8: 440–447
50. Faden AI (1984) Opiate antagonists in the treatment of stroke. Stroke 15: 575–578
51. Farhat SM, Schneider RC (1967) Observations on the effect of systemic blood pressure on intracranial circulation in patients with cerebrovascular insufficiency. J Neurosurg 27: 441–445
52. Flamm ES (1980) Treatment of cerebral vasospasm with aminophylline and isoproterenol. In: Wilkins RH (ed) Cerebral arterial spasm. Williams & Wilkins, Baltimore London, pp 575–577
53. Flamm ES, Adams HP, Beck DW *et al* (1988) Dose-escalation study of intravenous nicardipine in patients with aneurysmal subarachnoid hemorrhage. J Neurosurg 68: 393–400
54. Flamm ES, Adams HP (1988) Intravenous nicardipine in patients with aneurysmal subarachnoid hemorrhage. In: Wilkins RH (ed) Cerebral vasospasm. Raven Press, New York, pp 495–502
55. Flamm ES, Ransohoff J (1976) Treatment of cerebral vasospasm by control of cyclic adenosine monophosphate. Surg Neurol 6: 223–226
56. Fleckenstein A (1983) History of calcium antagonists. Circ Res 52 [Suppl 1]: 3–16
57. Fleischer AG, Raggio JF, Tindall GT (1977) Aminophylline and isoproterenol in the treatment of cerebral vasospasm. Surg Neurol 8: 286–290
58. Fleischer AS, Tindall GT (1980) Cerebral vasospasm following aneurysm rupture: a protocol for therapy and prophylaxis. J Neurosurg 52: 149–152
59. Fodstad H (1982) Antifibrinolytic treatment in subarachnoid hemorrhage: present state. Acta Neurochir (Wien) 63: 233–244
60. Fodstad H, Forssell A, Lilequiest B *et al* (1978) Tranexamic acid in the preoperative management of ruptured intracranial aneurysms. Surg Neurol 10: 9–15
61. Fodstad H, Pilbrant A, Schannong M *et al* (1981) Determination of tranexamic acid and fibrin/fibrinogen degradation products in cerebrospinal fluid after aneurysmal subarachnoid hemorrhage. Acta Neurochir (Wien) 58: 1–13

62. Fox JL, Falik JL, Shalhoub RJ (1971) Neurosurgical hyponatremia: the role of inappropriate antidiuresis. J Neurosurg 34: 506–514
63. Frazee JG, Bevan JA, Bevan RD *et al* (1988) Early treatment with diltiazem reduces delayed cerebral vascular narrowing after subarachnoid hemorrhage. Neurosurgery 23: 611–615
64. Frazee JG, Bevan JA, Bevan RD *et al* (1985) Effect of diltiazem on experimental chronic cerebral vasospasm in the monkey. J Neurosurg 62: 912–917
65. Fujita S, Kawaguchi T, Shose Y *et al.* (1990) Flunarizine treatment in poor-grade aneurysm patients. Acta Neurochir (Wien) 103: 11–17
66. George B, Muzard O, Begue T *et al* (1984) Efficacité d'un traitement médical (isoprotérénol + aminophylline) du spasme des ruptures anévrysmales. Neurochirurgie 30: 273–276
67. Giannotta SL, McGillicudy JE, Kindt GW (1977) Diagnosis and treatment of postoperative vasospasm. Surg Neurol 8: 286–290
68. Gilsbach JM (1988) Nimodipine in the prevention of ischaemic deficits after aneurysmal subarachnoid hemorrhage. An analysis of recent clinical studies. In: Reulen HJ, Philippon J (eds) Prevention and treatment of delayed ischaemic dysfunction in patients with subarachnoid hemorrhage. Acta Neurochir (Wien) [Suppl] 45. Springer, Wien New York, pp 41–50
69. Gilsbach JM, Harders AG (1989) Morbidity and mortality after early aneurysm surgery — a prospective study with nimodipine prevention. Acta Neurochir (Wien) 96: 1–7
70. Glick R, Green D, Ts'ao CH *et al* (1981) High-dose e-aminocaproïc acid prolongs the bleeding time and increases rebleeding and intraoperative hemorrhage in patients with subarachnoid hemorrhage. Neurosurgery 9: 398–401
71. Goetz KL (1988) Physiology and pathophysiology of atrial peptides. Am J Physiol 254: E1–E15
72. Gottstein U, Paulson OB (1972) The effect of intracarotid aminophylline infusion on the cerebral circulation. Stroke 3: 560–565
73. Grotenhuis JA, Bettag W, Fiebach BJO *et al* (1984) Intracarotid slow bolus injection of nimodipine during angiography for treatment of cerebral vasospasm. J Neurosurg 61: 231–240
74. Grotta JC (1987) Current status of hemodilution in acute cerebral ischemia. Stroke 18: 689–690
75. Grubb RL, Raichle ME, Eichling JO *et al* (1977) Effects of subarachnoid hemorrhage on cerebral blood volume, blood flow and oxygen utilization in humans. J Neurosurg 46: 446–453
76. Haraguchi S, Ebina K (1982) Evaluation of the dopamine induced hypertension therapy for vasospasm. Neurol Surg 10: 279–282
77. Harper AM, Craigen L, Kasda S (1981) Effect of calcium antagonist, nimodipine, on cerebral blood flow and metabolism in the primate. J Cereb Blood Flow Metab 1: 349–356
78. Hart RG, Byer JA, Slaughter JR *et al* (1981) Occurrence and implications of seizures in subarachnoid hemorrhage due to ruptured intracranial aneurysms. Neurosurgery 8: 417–421

79. Hasan D, Lindsay KW, Widjicks EFM *et al* (1989) Effect of fludrocortisone acetate in patients with subarachnoid hemorrhage. Stroke 20: 1156–1161
80. Hasan D, Vermeulen M, Wijdicks EFM *et al* (1989) Effect of fluid intake and hypertensive treatment on cerebral ischemia after subarachnoid hemorrhage. Stroke 20: 1511–1515
81. Hashi K, Matsuoka Y, Matsumoto Y *et al* (1980) Treatment of cerebral vasospasm with large doses of hydrocortisone. In: Wilkins RH (ed) Cerebral arterial spasm. Williams & Wilkins, Baltimore London, pp 611–618
82. Hashi K, Tabaka K (1980) Barbiturate coma for severe brain ischemia due to cerebral vasospasm. In: Wilkins RH (ed) Cerebral arterial spasm. Williams & Wilkins, Baltimore London, pp 637–645
83. The Hemodilution in Stroke Study Group (1989) Hypervolemic hemodilution treatment of acute stroke: results of a randomized multicentric trial using Pentastarch. Stroke 20: 317–323
84. Heros RC, Korosue K (1989) Hemodilution for cerebral ischemia. Stroke 20: 423–427
85. Higuchi S, Shiobara Y (1980) Comparative pharmacokinetics of nicardipine hypochloride, a new vasodilator, in various species. Xenobiotica 10: 447–454
86. Hijdra A, Vermeulen M, van Gijn J *et al* (1984) Respiratory arrest in subarachnoid hemorrhage. Neurology 34: 1501–1503
87. Hillman J, v. Essen C, Lezniewski W (1988) Results of treatment for cerebral saccular aneurysms in a small neurosurgical unit. Evaluation of early operation and nimodipine treatment. Acta Neurochir (Wien) 94: 28–31
88. Hino A, Mizukawa N, Tenjin H *et al* (1989) Postoperative hemodynamic and metabolic changes in patients with subarachnoid hemorrhage. Stroke 20: 1504–1510
89. Höllerhage HG, Gaab MR, Zumkeller M *et al* (1988) The influence of nimodipine on cerebral blood flow autoregulation and blood-brain barrier. J Neurosurg 69: 919–922
90. Italian Acute Stroke Study Group (1988) Haemodilution in acute stroke: results of the Italian haemodilution trial. The Lancet 13: 318–321
91. Jan M, Buchheit F, Tremoulet M (1988) Therapeutic trial of intravenous nimodipine in patients with established cerebral vasospasm after rupture of intracranial aneurysms. Neurosurgery 23: 154–157
92. Joynt RJ, Afifi A, Hardison J (1965) Hyponatremia in subarachnoid hemorrhage. Arch Neurol 13: 633–638
93. Kapp J, Neill WR, Salter JE *et al* (1987) Systemic heparin in the early management of ruptured intracranial aneurysms: review of 104 consecutive cases and comparison with concurrent controls. Neurosurgery 20: 564–570
94. Kapp JP, Clower BR, Azar FM *et al* (1985) Heparin reduces proliferative angiopathy following subarachnoid hemorrhage in cats. J Neurosurg 62: 570–575
95. Kassell NF, Peerless SJ, Drake CG *et al* (1980) Treatment of ischemic deficits from cerebral vasospasm with high dose barbiturate therapy. Neurosurgery 7: 593–597

96. Kassell NF, Peerless SJ, Durward QJ *et al* (1982) Treatment of ischemic deficits from vasospasm with intravascular volume expansion and induced arterial hypertension. Neurosurgery 11: 337–343
97. Kassell NF, Saski T, Colohan ART *et al* (1985) Cerebral vasospasm following aneurysmal subarachnoid hemorrhage. Stroke 16: 562–572
98. Kassell NF, Torner JC, Adams HP Jr. (1984) Antifibrinolytic therapy in the acute period following aneurysmal subarachnoid hemorrhage: Preliminary observations from the cooperative aneurysm study. J Neurosurg 61: 225–230
99. Kaye AH, Brownbill D (1981) Postoperative intracranial pressure in patients operated on for cerebral aneurysms following subarachnoid hemorrhage. J Neurosurg 54: 726–732
100. Kazda S (1985) Pharmacology of nimodipine, a calcium antagonist with preferential cerebrovascular activity. Neurochirurgia 28: 70–73
101. Kazda S, Towart R (1981) Differences of the calcium antagonist nimodipine (BAY e 9736) and bencyclan on cerebral and peripheral vascular smooth muscle. Br J Pharmacol 72: 582–583
102. Keränen T, Tapaninaho A, Hernesniemi J *et al* (1985) Late epilepsy after aneurysms operations. Neurosurgery 17: 897–900
103. Kim DS, Kang JK, Song JU (1989) Flunarizine treatment in SAH patients. Session on Cerebrovascular Disorders: 9th International Congress of Neurological Surgery, pp Abstract 103056, p 63
104. Kindt GW, McGilliculdy J, Pritz M *et al* (1980) Hypertension and hypervolemia as therapy for patients with vasospasm. In: Wilkins RH (ed) Cerebral arterial spasm. Williams and Wilkins, Baltimore, pp 661–668.
105. Kita H, Shima K, Akiya I *et al* (1989) Hemorrheological effects of ticlopidine in the treatment of cerebral vasospasm after subarachnoid hemorrhage. Session on Cerebrovascular Disorders: 9th International Congress of Neurological Surgery, pp Abstract 103059, p 64
106. Knuckey NW, Stokes BAR (1982) Medical management of patients following a ruptured cerebral aneurysm with e-aminocaproïc acid, kanamycine, and reserpine. Surg Neurol 17: 181–185
107. Koos WT, Perneczky A, Auer LM *et al* (1985) Nimodipine treatment of ischemic neurological deficits due to cerebral vasospasm after subarachnoid hemorrhage: clinical results of a multicenter study. Neurochirurgia (Stuttg) 28: 114–117
108. Kosnik EJ, Hunt WE (1976) Postoperative hypertension in the management of patients with intracranial arterial aneurysms. J Neurosurg 45: 148–154
109. Laine E, Bousquet C, Parquet-Gernez A (1978) Intérêt du bilan sanguin lipido-glucidique d'une part, de l'étude des fonctions plaquettaires d'autre part, dans la conduite du traitement des anévrysmes artériels intracrâniens. Neurochirurgie 24: 239–246
110. Lester M, Nelson PB (1981) Neurological aspects of vasopressin release and the syndrome of inappropriate secretion of antidiuretic hormone. Neurosurgery 8: 735–740

111. Levy WJ, Bay JW, Sawhny B *et al* (1982) Aminophylline plus nitroprusside and dopamine for treatment of cerebral vasospasm: a preliminary report. J Neurosurg 56: 646–649
112. Lindsay KW (1987) Antifibrinolytic agents in subarachnoid hemorrhage. J Neurol 234: 1–8
113. Ljunggren B, Brandt L, Saveland H *et al* (1984) Outcome in 60 consecutive patients treated with early aneurysm operation and intravenous nimodipine. J Neurosurg 62: 864–873
114. Loeb HS, Khan M, Saudye A *et al* (1976) Acute hemodynamic effects of dobutamide and isoproterenol in patients with low cardiac failure. Circ Shock 3: 55–63
115. Marin J, Lobato RD, Rico ML *et al* (1981) Effect of pentobarbital on the reactivity of isolated human cerebral arteries. J Neurosurg 54: 521–524
116. Marion DW, Segal R, Thompson ME (1986) Subarachnoid hemorrhage and the heart. Neurosurgery 18: 101–106
117. Maroon JC, Nelson PB (1979) Hypovolemia in patients with subarachnoid hemorrhage: therapeutic implications. Neurosurgery 4: 223–226
118. Martin WRW, Baker RP, Grubb RL *et al* (1984) Cerebral blood volume, blood flow, and oxygen metabolism in cerebral ischemia and subarachnoid hemorrhage: an in-vivo study using positron emission tomography. Acta Neurochir (Wien) 70: 3–9
119. Maurice-Williams RS, Gordon YB, Sykes A (1980) Monitoring fibrinolytic activity in the cerebrospinal fluid after aneurysmal subarachnoid hemorrhage: a guide to the risk of rebleeding? J Neurol Neurosurg Psychiatry 43: 175–181
120. Mee EW, Dorrance DE, Lowe D *et al* (1988) Controlled study of nimodipine in aneurysm patients treated early after subarachnoid hemorrhage. Neurosurgery 22: 484–491
121. Mendelow AD, Dharker S, Patterson J *et al* (1986) The dopamine withdrawal test following surgery for intracranial aneurysms. J Neurol Neurosurg Psychiatry 49: 35–38
122. Messeter K, Brandt L, Ljunggren B *et al* (1987) Prediction and prevention of delayed ischemic dysfunction after aneurysmal subarachnoid hemorrhage and early operation. Neurosurgery 20: 548–553
123. Miyagi K, Ishijima B, Sato F *et al* (1984) Indication for the method of and result of the prophylactic use of barbiturate therapy (B-therapy) against cerebral infarct from cerebral arterial vasospasm due to ruptured aneurysm. Neurol Surg 12: 303–310
124. Montgomery EB, Grubb RL, Raichle ME (1981) Cerebral hemodynamics and metabolism in postoperative cerebral vasospasm and treatment with hypertensive therapy. Ann Neurol 9: 502–506
125. Muizelaar JP, Becker DP (1986) Induced hypertension for the treatment of cerebral ischemia after subarachnoid hemorrhage. Surg Neurol 25: 317–325
126. Muizelaar JP, Wei EP, Kontos HA *et al* (1986) Cerebral blood flow is regulated by changes in blood pressure and in blood viscosity alike. Stroke 17: 44–48

127. Mullan S, Beckman F, Vailati G *et al* (1964) An experimental approach to the problem of cerebral aneurysms. J Neurosurg 21: 838–845
128. Mullan S, Dawley J (1968) Antifibrinolytic therapy for intracranial aneurysms. J Neurosurg 28: 21–23
129. Neil-Dwyer G, Cruishank J, Stratton C (1986) β-blockers, plasma total creatinine kinase and creatinine kinase myocardial isoenzyme, and the prognosis of subarachnoid hemorrhage. Drugs 25: 163–168
130. Neil-Dwyer G, Walter P, Cruishank J *et al* (1983) β-Blockade in subarachnoid hemorrhage. Drugs 25 [Suppl 2]: 273–277
131. Nelson PB, Seif S, Gutai J *et al* (1984) Hypoatremia with natriuresis following subarachnoid hemorrhage in a monkey model. J Neurosurg 60: 233–237
132. Nelson PB, Seif SM, Maroon JC *et al* (1981) Hyponatremia in intracranial disease: perhaps not the syndrome of inappropriate secretion of antidiuretic hormone. J Neurosurg 55: 938–941
133. Nibbelink DW, Torner JC, Henderson WC (1975) Intracranial aneurysms and subarachnoid hemorrhage. A cooperative study. Antifibrinolytic therapy in recent onset subarachnoid hemorrhage. Stroke 6: 622–629
134. Norlen G, Thulin CA (1969) The use of antifibrinolytic substance in ruptured intracranial aneurysms. Neurochirurgia (Stuttg) 12: 100–102
135. North JB, Penhall RK, Hanieh A *et al* (1983) Phenytoin and postoperative epilepsy. J Neurosurg 58: 672–677
136. Nosko M, Schulz R, Weir B *et al* (1988) Effects of vasospasm on levels of prostacyclin and thromboxane A2. Neurosurgery 22: 45–50
137. Nosko M, Weir B, Krueger C *et al* (1985) Nimodipine and chronic vasospasm in monkeys: Part 1. Clinical and radiological findings. Neurosurgery 16: 129–136
138. Ochiai C, Asano T, Takakura K (1982) Mechanisms of cerebral protection by pentobarbital and nizofenone correlated with the course of local cerebral blood flow changes. Stroke 13: 788–796
139. Öhman J, Heiskanen O (1988) Effect of nimodipine on the outcome of patients after aneurysmal subarachnoid hemorrhage and surgery. J Neurosurg 69: 683–686
140. Öhman J, Heiskanen O (1989) Timing of operation for ruptured supratentorial aneurysms: a prospective randomized study. J Neurosurg 70: 55–60
141. Olesen J, Hougard K, Hertz M (1978) Isoproterenol and propanolol: ability to cross the blood-brain barrier and effects on cerebral circulation in man. Stroke 9: 344-349
142. Park BE (1979) Spontaneous subarachnoid hemorrhage complicated by communicating hydrocephalus: an aminocaproïc acid as a possible predisposing factor. Surg Neurol 11: 73–80
143. Petruk KC, West M, Mohr G *et al* (1988) Nimodipine treatment in the poorgrade aneurysm patients: results of a multicentre double-blind placebo-controlled trial. J Neurosurg 68: 505–517
144. Philippon J, Grob R, Dagreon F *et al* (1986) Prevention of vasospasm in subarachnoid hemorrhage. A controlled study with nimodipine. Acta Neurochir (Wien) 82: 110–114

145. Pickard JD, Murray GD, Illingworth R *et al* (1989) Effect of oral nimodipine on cerebral infarction and outcome after subarachnoid hemorrhage: British aneurysm nimodipine trial. Br Med J 298: 636–642
146. Poungvarin N, Bhoopat W, Viriyavejakul A *et al* (1987) Effects of dexamethasone in primary supratentorial intracerebral hemorrhage. N Engl J Med 316: 1229–1233
147. Pritz MB, Giannotta SL, Kindt GW *et al* (1978) Treatment of patients with neurological deficits associated with cerebral vasospasm by intravascular volume expansion. Neurosurgery 3: 364–368
148. Quirion R (1988) Atrial natriuretic factors and the brain: an update. Trends Neurosci 11: 58–62
149. Ramirez-Lassepas M (1981) Antifibrinolytic therapy in subarachnoid hemorrhage caused by ruptured intracranial aneurysm. Neurology 31: 316–322
150. Rämsch KD, Ahr G, Tettenborn D *et al* (1985) Overview on pharmacokinetics of nimodipine in healthy volunteers and in patients with subarachnoid hemorrhage. Neurochirurgia 28: 74–78
151. Reeder RF, Harbaugh RE (1989) Administration of intravenous urea and normal saline for the treatment of hyponatremia in neurosurgical patients. J Neurosurg 70: 201–206
152. Ritchie WI, Weir B, Overton TR (1980) Experimental subarachnoid hemorrhage in the cynomolgus monkey: evaluation of treatment with hypertension, volume expansion, and ventilation. Neurosurgery 6: 57–62
153. Rodriguez y Baena R, Gaetani P, Marzatico MS *et al* (1989) Effects of Nicardipine on the ex vivo release of eicosanoïds after experimental subarachnoid hemorrhage. J Neurosurg 71: 903–908
154. Rosenfeld JV, Barnett GH, Sila CA *et al* (1989) The effect of subarachnoid hemorrhage on blood and CSF atrial natriuretic factor. J Neurosurg 71: 32–37
155. Rosenwasser RH, Delgado TE, Bucheit WA *et al* (1983) Control of hypertension and prophylaxis against vasospasm in cases of subarachnoid hemorrhage: a preliminary report. Neurosurgery 12: 658–661
156. Rudehill A, Olsson GL, Sundqvist K *et al* (1987) ECG abnormalities in patients with subarachnoid hemorrhage and intracranial tumors. J Neurol Neurosurg Psychiatry 50: 1375–1381
157. Saito I, Asano T, Ochiai C *et al* (1983) A double-blind clinical evaluation of the effect of Nizofenone (Y-9179) on delayed ischemic neurological deficits following aneurysmal rupture. Neurol Res 5: 29–47
158. Samson DS, Beyer CM (1980) Thiopental coma in the treatment of vasospasm-induced cerebral ischemia/infarction. In: Wilkins RH (ed) Cerebral arterial spasm. Williams & Wilkins, Baltimore London, pp 634–645
159. Saunders FW (1986) Diltiazem: possible hematologic complications. Surg. Neurol 25: 82–84
160. Säveland H, Ljunggren B, Brandt L *et al* (1986) Delayed ischemic deterioration in patients with early aneurysm operation and intravenous nimodipine. Neurosurgery 18: 146–150
161. Sawaya R, Sonnino V, McLaurin RL *et al* (1983) Monitoring of antifibrinolytic therapy following subarachnoid hemorrhage. The importance of CSF fibrin/fibrinogen degradation products. J Neurosurg 58: 699–707

162. Sbeih I, Tamas LB, O'Laoire SA (1986) Epilepsy after operation for aneurysms. Neurosurgery 19: 784–788
163. Schwartz WB, Bennett W, Curelop S, Bartter FC (1957) A syndrome of renal sodium loss and hyponatremia probably resulting from inappropriate secretion of antidiuretic hormone. Am J Med 23: 529–542
164. Seiler RW, Reulen HJ, Huber P *et al* (1988) Outcome of aneurysmal subarachnoid hemorrhage in a hospital population: a prospective study including early operation, intravenous nimodipine, transcranial doppler. Neurosurgery 23: 598–604
165. Shaw MDM, Foy PM, Huber P *et al* (1985) Dipyridamole and postoperative ischemic deficits in aneurysmal subarachnoid hemorrhage. J Neurosurg 63: 699–703
166. Shimoda M, Yamada S, Yamamoto I *et al* (1989) Atrial natriuretic polypeptide in patients with subarachnoid hemorrhage due to aneurysmal rupture. Acta Neurochir (Wien) 97: 53–61
167. Siesjö BK (1984) Cerebral circulation and metabolism. J Neurosurg 60: 883–908
168. Singh BN (1986) The mechanism of action of calcium antagonists relative to their clinical applications. Br J Clin Pharmacol 21: 109S–121S
169. Solomon RA, Fink ME, Lennihan L (1988) Early aneurysm surgery and prophylactic hypervolemic hypertensive therapy for the treatment of aneurysmal subarachnoid hemorrhage. Neurosurgery 23: 699–704
170. Solomon RA, Post KD, McMurty JG III (1984) Depression of circulating blood volume in patients after subarachnoid hemorrhage: implications for the management of symptomatic vasospasm. Neurosurgery 15: 354–361
171. Sonnenblick EH, Frishman WH, Le Jemtel TH (1979) Dobutamide: a new synthetic cardioactive sympathetic amine. N Engl J Med 300: 17–21
172. Stober T, Anstätt Th, Sen S *et al* (1988) Cardiac arrhythmias in subarachnoid hemorrhage. Acta Neurochir (Wien) 93: 37–44
173. Sundt TM (1975) Management of ischemic complications after subarachnoid hemorrhage. J Neurosurg 43: 418–425
174. Sundt TM, Onofrio BM, Merideth J (1973) Treatment of cerebral vasospasm from subarachnoid hemorrhage with isoproterenol and lidocaïne hydrochloride. J Neurosurg 38: 557–559
175. Suzuki S, Iwabuchi T, Tanaka T *et al* (1985) Prevention of cerebral vasospasm with OKY-046, an imidazole derivative and a thromboxane syntetase inhibitor. A preliminary co-operative clinical study. Acta Neurochir (Wien) 77: 133–141
176. Suzuki S, Sobata E, Iwabuchi T (1981) Prevention of cerebral ischemic symptoms in cerebral vasospasm with Trapidil, an antagonist and selective synthesis inhibitor of thromboxane A2. Neurosurgery 9: 679–685
177. Symon L (1980) General conclusions: suggestions for further research. In: Wilkins RH (ed) Cerebral arterial spasm. Williams & Wilkins, Baltimore London, pp 693–694
178. Tabbaa MA, Ramirez-Lassepas M, Snyder BD (1987) Aneurysmal subarachnoid hemorrhage presenting as cardiorespiratory arrest. Arch Intern Med 147: 1661-1662

179. Takaku A, Shindo K, Tanaka S *et al* (1979) Fluid and electrolyte disturbances in patients with intracranial aneurysms. Surg Neurol 11: 349–356
180. Takenaka T, Handa J (1979) Cerebrovascular effects of YC-93, a new vasodilator, in dogs, monkeys and human patients. Int J Clin Pharmacol Biopharm 17: 1–11
181. Takeuchi S, Koike T, Sasaki O *et al* (1989) Intracranial extradural pressure monitoring after direct operation on ruptured cerebral aneurysms. Neurosurgery 24: 878–883
182. Tanabe T, Lewis PJ, Itoh H *et al* (1988) Hypervolemic therapy without induced hypertension in patients with severe subarachnoid hemorrhage. In: Wilkins RH (ed) Cerebral vasospasm. Raven Press, New York, pp 421–424
183. Tanabe T, Saitoh T, Tachibana S *et al* (1982) Effect of hyperdynamic therapy on cerebral ischemia caused by vasospasm associated with subarachnoid hemorrhage. Acta Neurochir (Wien) 63: 291–296
184. Tani E, Maeda Y, Fukumori T *et al* (1984) Effect of selective inhibitor of thromboxane A2 synthetase on cerebral vasospasm after early surgery. J Neurosurg 61: 24–29
185. Tsementzis SA, Hitchcock ER, Meyer CHA (1990) Benefits and risks of antifibrinolytic therapy in the management of ruptured intracranial aneurysms. Acta Neurochir (Wien) 102: 1–10
186. Van Breeman C, Hwang OK, Meisheri KD (1981) The mechanism of inhibitory action of diltiazem on vascular smooth muscle contractility. J Pharmacol Exp Ther 218: 459–463
187. VanderArk GD, Pomerantz M (1973) Reversal of ischemic neurological signs by increasing the cardiac output. Surg Neurol 1: 257–258
188. Varsos VG, Liszciak TM, Hee Han D *et al* (1983) Delayed cerebral vasospasm is not reversible by aminophylline, nifedipine or papaverine in a "two hemorrhage" canine model. J Neurosurg 58: 11–17
189. Vasu MA, O'Keefe DD, Kapellakis GZ *et al* (1978) Myocardial oxygen consumption: effects of epinephrine, isoproterenol, dopamine, norepinephrine, and dobutamine. Am J Physiol 235: H237–H241
190. Vermeulen M, Lindsay KW, Murray GD *et al* (1984) Antifibrinolytic treatment in subarachnoid hemorrhage. N Engl J Med 311: 432–437
191. Vermeulen M, van Vliet HHDM, Lindsay KW *et al* (1985) Source of fibrin/fibrinogen degradation products in the CSF after subarachnoid hemorrhage. J Neurosurg 63: 573–577
192. Vinge E, Brandt L, Ljunggren B *et al* (1988) Thromboxane B2 levels in serum during continuous administration of nimodipine to patients with aneurysmal subarachnoid hemorrhage. Stroke 19: 644–647
193. Voldby B, Enevoldsen EM, Jensen FT (1985) Cerebrovascular reactivity in patients with ruptured intracranial aneurysms. J Neurosurg 62: 59–67
194. Voldby B, Enevoldsen EM, Jensen FT (1985) Regional CBF, intraventricular pressure, and cerebral metabolism in patients with ruptured intracranial aneurysms. J Neurosurg 62: 48–58
195. von Essen C, Zervas NT, Brown DR *et al* (1980) Local cerebral blood flow in the dog during intravenous infusion of dopamine. Surg Neurol 13: 181–188

196. Weinand ME, O'Boynick OL, Goetz KL (1989) A study of serum antidiuretic hormone and atrial natriuretic peptide levels in a series of patients with intracranial disease and hyponatremia. Neurosurgery 25: 781–785
197. Weir B (1987) Antifibrinolytics in subarachnoid hemorrhage. Do they have a role? No. Arch Neurol 44: 116–118
198. White RP, Robertson JT (1987) Pharmacodynamic evaluation of human cerebral arteries in the genesis of vasospasm. Neurosurgery 21: 523–531
199. Wijdicks EFM, Hasan D, Lindsay KW *et al* (1989) Short-term tranexamic acid treatment in aneurysmal subarachnoid hemorrhage. Stroke 20: 1674–1679
200. Wijdicks EFM, Vermeulen M, Hijdra A *et al* (1985) Hyponatremia and cerebral infarction in patients with ruptured intracranial aneurysms: is fluid restriction harmful? Ann Neurol 17: 137–140
201. Wilkins RH (1986) Attempts at the prevention or treatment of intracranial arterial spasm: an update. Neurosurgery 18: 808–825
202. Winn HR, Richardson AE, O'Brien W *et al* (1978) The long-term prognosis in untreated cerebral aneurysms. Ann Neurol 4: 418–426
203. Wise BL (1978) Syndrome of inappropriate antidiuretic hormone secretion after spontaneous subarachnoid hemorrhage: a reversible cause of clinical deterioration. Neurosurgery 3: 412–414
204. Wood JH, Simeone FA, Kron RE *et al* (1984) Experimental hypervolemic hemodilution: physiological correlations of cortical blood flow, cardiac output, and intracranial pressure with fresh blood viscosity and plasma volume. Neurosurgery 14: 709–723
205. Wood JH, Simeone FA, Fink EA *et al* (1983) Hypervolemic hemodilution in experimental focal cerebral ischemia. Elevation of cardiac output, regional cortical blood flow, and ICP after intravascular volume expansion with low molecular weight dextran. J Neurosurg 59: 500–509
206. Wood JH, Simeone FA, Kron RE *et al* (1982) Rheological aspects of experimental hypervolemic hemodilution with low molecular weight Dextran: relationships of cortical blood flow, cardiac output, and intracranial pressure to fresh blood viscosity and plasma volume. Neurosurgery 11: 739–753
207. Wood JH, Snyder LL, Simeone FA (1982) Failure of intravascular volume expansion without hemodilution to elevate cortical blood flow in region of experimental focal ischemia. J Neurosurg 56: 80–91
208. Yamakami I, Isobe K, Yamaura A (1987) Effects of intravascular volume expansion on cerebral blood flow in patients with ruptured cerebral aneurysms. Neurosurgery 21: 303–309
209. Yamamoto M, Ohta T, Toda N (1983) Mechanisms of relaxant action of nicardipine, a new Ca++ antagonist, on isolated dog cerebral and mesenteric arteries. Stroke 14: 270–275
210. Yamaura A, Nakamura T, Makino H *et al* (1980) Cerebral complication of antifibrinolytic therapy in the treatment of ruptured intracranial aneurysm. Animal experiment and a review of literature. Eur Neurol 19: 77–84
211. Yonas H, Sekhar L, Johnson DW *et al* (1989) Determination of irreversible ischemia by Xenon-enhanced computed tomographic monitoring of cerebral blood flow in patients with symptomatic vasospasm. Neurosurgery 24: 368–372

212. Young B, Rapp RP, Norton JA *et al* (1983) Failure of prophylactically administered phenytoin to prevent late posttraumatic seizures. J Neurosurg 58: 236–241
213. Zervas NT, Candia M, Candia G *et al* (1979) Reduced incidence of cerebral ischemia following rupture of intracranial aneurysms. Surg Neurol 11: 339–344
214. Zervas NT, Kistler JP, Ploetz J (1980) Effect of reserpine and kanamycin on postoperative delayed ischemic deficits in patients with subarachnoid hemorrhage after aneurysmal rupture. In: Wilkins RH (ed) Cerebral arterial spasm. Williams & Wilkins, Baltimore London, pp 514–517

B. Technical Standards

Unilateral Partial Hemilaminectomy for the Removal of Extra- and Intramedullary Tumours and AVMs

M. G. Yaşargil, B. I. Tranmer*, T. E. Adamson, and P. Roth

Department of Neurosurgery, University of Zürich, Zürich (Switzerland) and
* Division of Neurosurgery, University of Calgary, Calgary (Canada)

With 9 Figures

Contents

In 1967, microsurgical techniques were introduced in Zürich. Since that time, the senior author has had the opportunity to operate on 78 spinal AVMs and 250 spinal tumours (46 extradural, 94 extramedullary, and 110 intramedullary tumours).

Extensive laminectomies have been advocated for the removal of spinal cord tumours since Horsley first removed a benign spinal cord tumour in 1887[13]. The first successful laminectomy was performed in 1829 by Alban Smith[18] and the modern approach to laminectomy is well described by Love[17]. The bilateral approach to the spinal cord has been recommended for years because it was believed that only such an approach would allow full visualization of the spinal cord and its relationship to spinal cord tumours. The current techniques of approach used for the removal of these lesions are the result of an attempt to minimize postoperative complications concerning the stability of the vertebral column. Initially, the main surgical objective was resection of the lesion without injury to the spinal cord, nerve

Table 1. *Microsurgical Treatment of Spinal Tumours (1967—1989)*

	Total	Cervical	Cervico-thoracal	Thoracal	Thoracolumbar	Lumbar	Lumbosacral	Sacral
Meningioma	33 (22)	7 (3)	–	21 (17)	2 (1)	2 (1)	1 (–)	–
Neurinoma	31 (12)	19 (9)	–	3 (1)	–	8 (2)	1 (–)	–
Ependymoma	40 (15)	11 (6)	14 (4)	7 (1)	7 (3)	1 (1)	–	–
Astrozytoma	31 (11)	15 (6)	4 (2)	12 (3)	–	–	–	–
Malignant glioma	2 (1)	–	1 (–)	1 (1)	–	–	–	–
Glioblastoma	2 (–)	–	–	2 (–)	–	–	–	–
Spongioblastoma	3 (–)	1 (–)	2 (–)	–	–	–	–	–
Angioblastoma	15 (5)	8 (3)	–	6 (1)	1 (1)	–	–	–
Cyst	6 (3)	1 (1)	–	2 (1)	2 (1)	–	–	1 (–)
Ganglioglioma	6 (2)	1 (1)	1 (–)	3 (1)	1 (–)	–	–	–
Angioglioma	1 (–)	–	1 (–)	–	–	–	–	–
Cavernoma	2 (2)	1 (1)	–	1 (1)	–	–	–	–
Lipoma	8 (3)	–	1 (1)	–	–	1 (–)	3 (1)	3 (1)
Angiolipoma	1 (–)	–	–	–	–	–	1 (–)	–
Dermoid	3 (2)	–	–	–	1 (–)	2 (2)	–	–
Teratoma	1 (–)	–	–	1 (–)	–	–	–	–
Sarcoma	7 (3)	3 (1)	–	1 (1)	1 (–)	1 (1)	–	1 (–)
Chordoma	5 (3)	–	1 (–)	3 (3)	1 (–)	–	–	–
Lymphoma	4 (1)	2 (1)	–	2 (–)	–	–	–	–
Thymoma	1 (1)	–	–	–	1 (1)	–	–	–
Wilms' tumor	1 (1)	–	–	–	1 (1)	–	–	–
Plasmocytoma	1 (–)	–	–	1 (–)	–	–	–	–
Aneurysm. bone cyst	1 (–)	–	–	1 (–)	–	–	–	–
Metastases	16 (4)	1 (–)	–	14 (4)	–	–	1 (–)	–
Medulloblastoma	5 (1)	1 (–)	1 (–)	–	3 (1)	–	–	–
Melanoma	7 (2)	1 (–)	–	4 (–)	2 (2)	–	–	–
Syringomyelia	8 (4)	7 (4)	1 (–)	–	–	–	–	–
Myelocele	2 (1)	–	1 (1)	–	–	–	1 (–)	–
Subarachn. cyst	3 (–)	1 (–)	–	1 (–)	–	–	1 (–)	–
Hematoma	2 (1)	–	1 (–)	1 (1)	–	–	–	–
Echinococcus	1 (–)	–	–	1 (–)	–	–	–	–
Tuberculosis	1 (–)	–	–	1 (–)	–	–	–	–
	250 (100)	80 (36)	29 (8)	89 (36)	23 (11)	15 (7)	9 (1)	5 (1)

( ) Operated since 1980.

Table 2. *Approaches to the Spinal Tumours (1967—1989)*

	Bilateral	Unilateral	Reconstructive	Total (1980–1989)
Cervical	52 (6)	(20)	(10)	(36)
Cervicothoracal	19 (4)	(2)	(2)	(8)
Thoracal	69 (16)	(16)	(4)	(36)
Thoracolumbar	12 (−)	(11)	(−)	(11)
Lumbar	15 (3)	(4)	(−)	(7)
Lumbosacral	9 (1)	(−)	(−)	(1)
Sacral	5 (1)	(−)	(−)	(1)
	181 (31)	(53)	(16)	(100) = 250

( ) Operated since 1980.

Table 3. *Localization of Tumours (1967—1989)*

	Extradural	Extramedullary	Intramedullary	Total
Cervical	7 (2)	28 (12)	45 (22)	80 (36)
Cervicothoracal	1 (−)	2 (−)	26 (8)	29 (8)
Thoracal	27 (8)	27 (18)	35 (10)	89 (36)
Thoracolumbar	6 (4)	13 (5)	4 (2)	23 (11)
Lumbar	3 (3)	12 (4)	−	15 (7)
Lumbosacral	1	8 (1)	−	9 (1)
Sacral	1	4 (1)	−	5 (1)
	46 (17)	94 (41)	110 (42)	250 (100)

( ) Cases operated since 1980.

roots or vascular structures. In patients with extra- or intramedullary tumours of relatively short length (1—4 cm), cervical, thoracic or lumbar laminectomies of 1—3 laminar segments caused at most minimal instability of the vertebral column. Long extending extra- or intramedullary tumours (5—20 cm), which required osteoplastic laminectomies along 5 to 15 laminar segments have not been without complications, especially in the case of children and young adults. Postlaminectomy vertebral column instability, severe kyphoscoliosis, spinal deformities, extradural scarring with dural constriction and loss of posterior osseous protection have all been described[3, 5, 14, 16, 19, 23, 24, 30].

Osteoplastic Laminectomy

The importance of the preservation of the posterior arch and its ligaments and paravertebral muscles has become more widely recognized and has led to the development of several new posterior approaches to the spinal cord[8, 10, 12, 20, 21, 25]. Our own experience with similar complications of spinal cord column stimulated us in 1973 to develop a technique to preserve the integrity of the posterior bony elements and soft tissues. It involves bilateral laminectomy with the help of an oscillating micro-saw which allows removal of the posterior arch (including spinal processes) in one piece. This is performed over several levels (3—6 or more) leaving the connecting ligamentous structures between the arches and processes intact. In cases in which radical removal of the tumour is possible and no postoperative swelling of the cord is anticipated the arches can be replaced. Two sutures at each end secure the laminae and the proximal and distal aspects are sutured to the adjacent ligamentous tissue. In 12 cervical and 4 thoracic intramedullary tumours this technique has been used successfully between 1973 and 1980. This osteoplastic laminectomy results in good stability of the spinal column but it was abandoned as a routine procedure since it requires immobilization of spinal column for at least 3 months during the healing and stabilization processes with resultant inconvenience to the patient and interference with necessary physiotherapy. In addition, when radical removal of an infiltrative intramedullary tumour was not possible, the laminae could not be replaced over the swollen cord.

Unilateral (Partial) Hemilaminectomy

Since 1980 the technique of more limited unilateral and partial hemilaminectomy has been developed. Microsurgical experiences with deep intracranial lesions have shown that they can be approached and removed without using wide exposure. Experience with microtechniques applied to disc surgery (lumbar, cervical or thoracic) and to surgery of small spinal meningiomas and neurinomas has proved convincingly that this limited hemilaminectomy is effective; such lesions could be successfully removed through a small one-sided opening in the soft tissue (skin and muscle) and with minimal resection of the bony elements.

Therefore we have adopted a similar approach also for extra- and intramedullary tumours. The unilateral approach and unilateral dissection of the paravertebral muscles, partial removal of 1—3 laminae, medial dural and arachnoidal openings provides visualization of both sides of the cord, even of contralateral nerves and vessels and enough space to dissect the tumour in a circumferential manner from both sides. Currently, meningiomas and neurinomas require only 1 or 1 ½ level hemilaminectomies whereas usually larger gliomas need partial unilateral resection of 3 to 6 laminae or more. The one-side approach saves the soft tissue of the opposite side, as well as the spinal process and the opposite lamina and ligament. Patients therefore can be mobilized the following day after surgery without the use of any external support.

The only tumours that are not removed by this approach are those which have extensive bilateral epidural invasion of the soft tissue surrounding the spinal cord. Intramedullary and extramedullary-intrathecal tumours at all spinal levels have been removed through this limited exposure of hemilaminectomy. The surgical exposure is illustrated in Fig. 3.

Clinical Material

In this series of 100 patients (since 1980), 101 spinal tumours (one patient had two neurinomas) have been resected by using the partial hemilaminectomy approach. The mean age of the 35 males and 65 females was 31 years (range 4—82). Tumours were removed from the cervical (36), cervicothoracic (8), thoracic (36), thoracolumbar (11), lumbar (7), lumbosacral (1) and sacral (1) regions (see Table 2). The average number of hemilaminectomies performed for each tumour was 4 (range 1—8). Seventeen tumours were epidural, 41 were extramedullary-intrathecal, and 42 were intramedullary (Table 3). The tumour pathology is detailed in Table 1. The commonest tumour removed was the intradural-extramedullary meningioma (33). The largest diameter tumour removed was a 5 cm diameter schwannoma located in the cervical region. The most extensive intramedullary tumour was an ependymoma extending from C2 to T6, and the most extensive epidural tumour was a metastatic chondrosarcoma extending from C7 to T4. In one patient with neurofibromatosis, two meningiomas were removed from the thoracic region and in addition a syringoperitoneal shunt was also performed through this exposure. No intraoperative complications (hemorrhage, spinal cord injury) were felt to have resulted from using this limited exposure. All patients have been carefully followed and no complications such as spinal deformity or spinal instability have been observed. Examples of the spinal cord tumours are shown in Figs. 6–8 (MRI and x-ray images).

Operative Technique

A lateral spinal x-ray is initially used to mark the surgical level for the removal of the spinal cord tumour (Fig. 1). With the patient in the prone position a paramedian skin incision is made on the side of tumours such as meningiomas, neurinomas or any other extramedullary lateral tumour. In the case of an intramedullary tumour, the extension of the tumour more to one side will dictate the side of approach. The subcutaneous tissue is incised to expose the dorsal fascia. The fascia is incised in a curvilinear

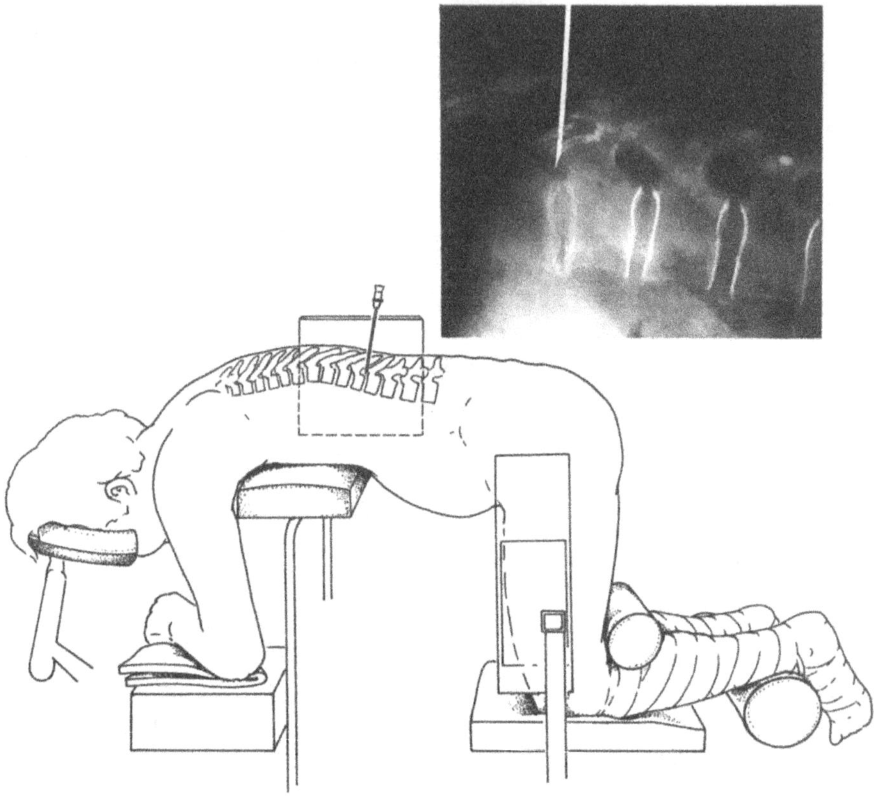

Fig. 1. The positioning of the patient for thoracic, and thoraco-lumbar spinal surgery; including a demonstration of the technique of level identification using a lateral x-ray and a spinal needle introduced at the target level

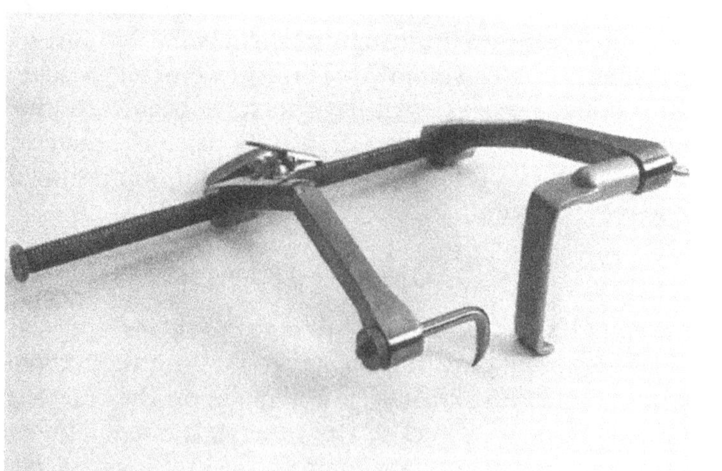

Fig. 2. The specially constructed self-retaining retractor used for unilateral hemi-laminectomies

fashion approximately 10 mm off the midline and reflected towards the midline leaving the intraspinal ligaments intact. The paravertebral muscles and ligaments on only one side of the spinous process are stripped subperiostally and reflected laterally. A specially constructed self-retaining retractor is used to maintain this exposure (Fig. 2). With the posterior spinal arch unilaterally exposed, a 6—8 mm wide hemilaminectomy is then performed using a high-speed electric drill and small Kerrison rongeurs. A small amount of bone may also be removed laterally with the rongeurs, but the joint is not removed. The spinous processes may be minimally undercut with the drill to gain access to the contralateral side. The bony opening is approximately 6—10 mm wide (Fig. 3). The ligamentum flavum

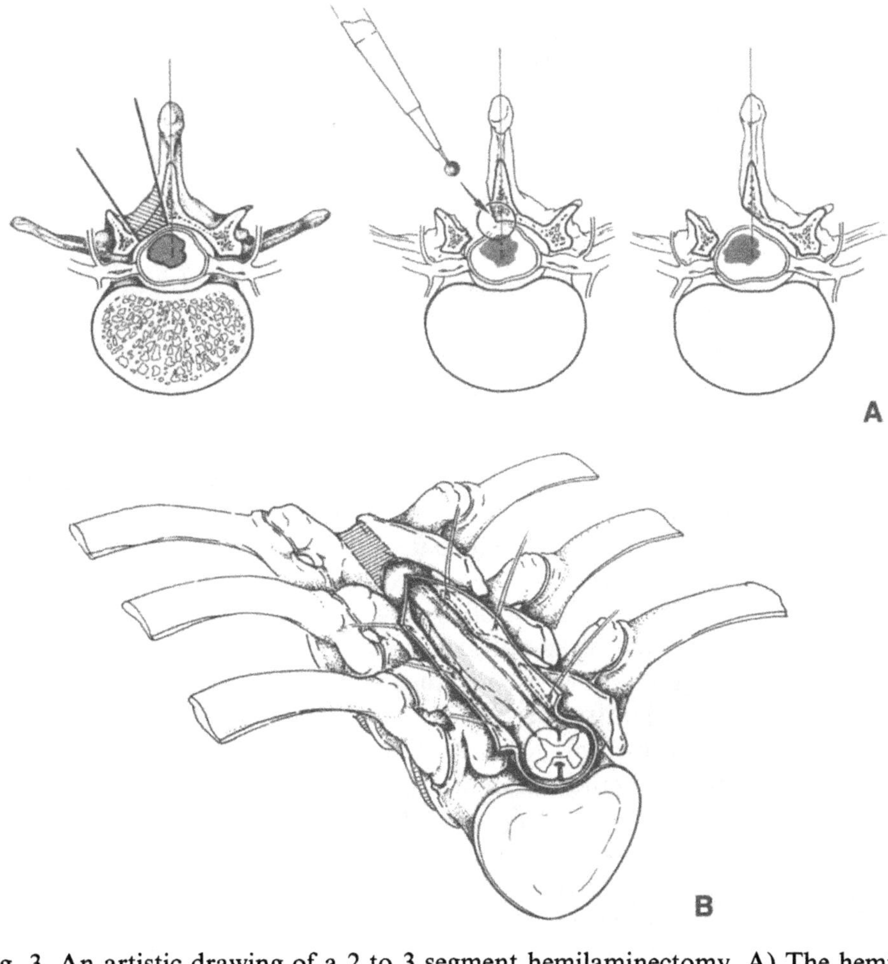

Fig. 3. An artistic drawing of a 2 to 3 segment hemilaminectomy. A) The hemilaminectomy and undermining of the spinous process using a high speed drill. B) Following the bone removal, the dura and arachnoid are opened in the midline with full dorsal visualization of the spinal cord

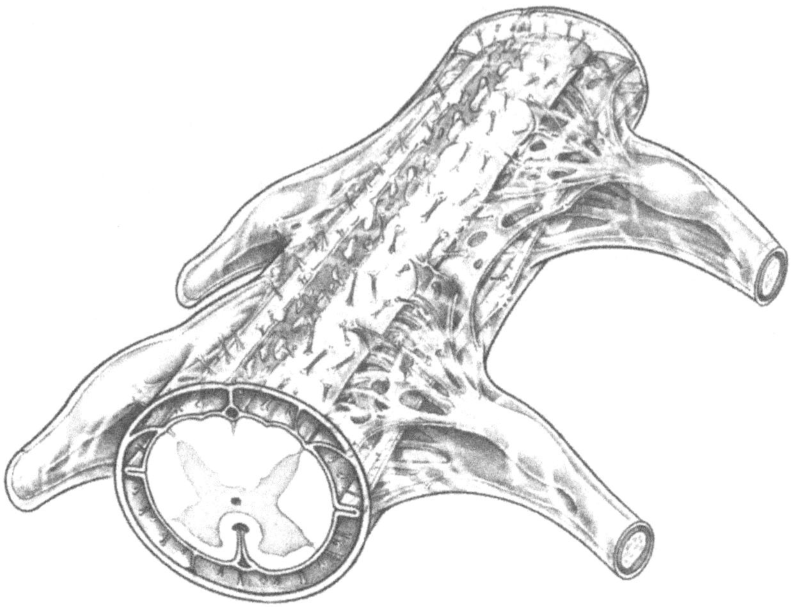

Fig. 4. An artistic drawing of the spinal cord and arachnoidal architecture. The midline septum which may be displaced by tumour expansion and pathological vessels is an important component of the arachnoidal covering

is then incised exposing the spinal dura. In the case of an intradural tumour, the dura is longitudinally incised in the midline. The arachnoid is also similarly opened and then reflected back, after cutting the numerous arachnoid fibers and arachnoidal septa in the dorsal midline, and secured to the edges of the dura with silver clips (Fig. 4).

By gently retracting the spinal cord and spinal roots, and adjusting the line of vision through the microscope, tumours can be removed from dorsal, dorsolateral, lateral, contralateral, ventral and dorsal aspects of the spinal cord. Extensive intramedullary tumours can also be resected through this approach after releasing the cyst in or around the tumour or decompression of the centre of the tumour and dissecting with the help of bipolar forceps around the tumour cleavage plane, sucking off the tumour piecemeal with the ultrasonic dissector (Cavitron).

Following tumour resection the arachnoid is reapproximated using bipolar thermo-coagulation or microsutures and then the dura is closed with a running suture (Fig. 5A–C). The fascia and skin are closed in the standard fashion. The muscles are not sutured. Representative cases are shown in Figs. 6—9.

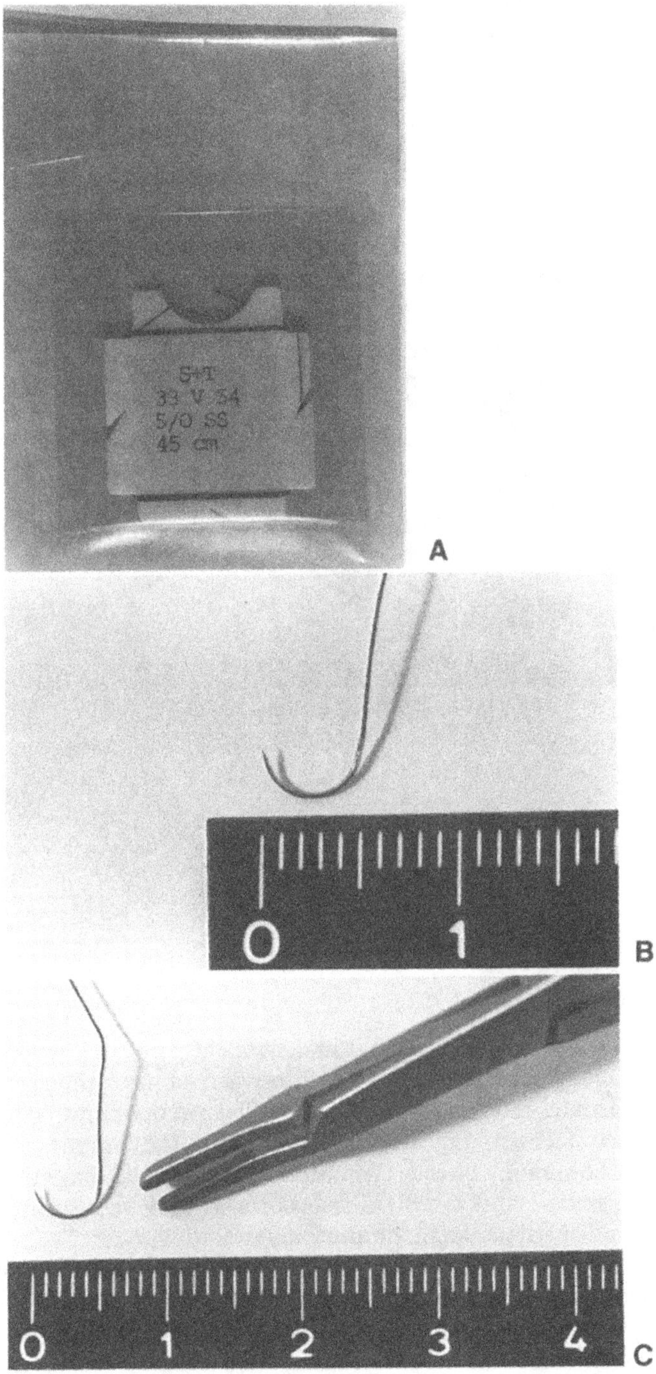

Fig. 5 A–C. Closure of the spinal dura through a hemilaminectomy required development of a new short radius needle. This needle is now commercially avalaible

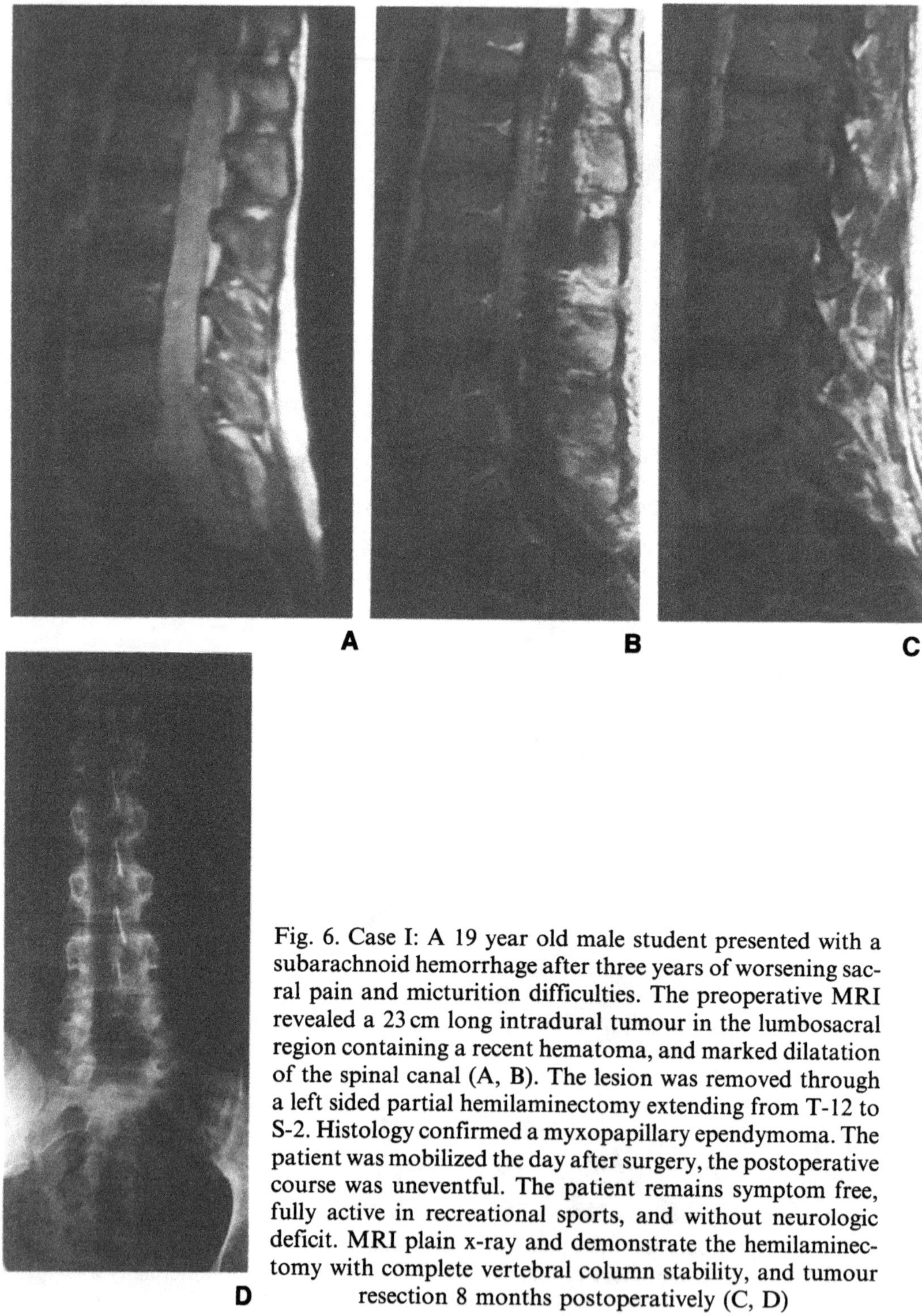

Fig. 6. Case I: A 19 year old male student presented with a subarachnoid hemorrhage after three years of worsening sacral pain and micturition difficulties. The preoperative MRI revealed a 23 cm long intradural tumour in the lumbosacral region containing a recent hematoma, and marked dilatation of the spinal canal (A, B). The lesion was removed through a left sided partial hemilaminectomy extending from T-12 to S-2. Histology confirmed a myxopapillary ependymoma. The patient was mobilized the day after surgery, the postoperative course was uneventful. The patient remains symptom free, fully active in recreational sports, and without neurologic deficit. MRI plain x-ray and demonstrate the hemilaminectomy with complete vertebral column stability, and tumour resection 8 months postoperatively (C, D)

Discussion

Although the standard multilevel laminectomy continues to be commonly used for spinal cord decompression, it may be associated with a number of postoperative complications. These problems, which include spinal deformity, spinal instability, dorsal extradural scar formation with dural constriction and absence of osseous protection for the spinal cord, may lead to a progressive myelopathy[3, 5, 14, 16, 19, 23, 24, 30].

Haft and associates were the first to describe the risk of kyphoscoliosis and instability after laminectomy for intraspinal tumour removal in children[11], and Bette and Engelhardt described in 1955 two adolescents who developed "swan-neck" deformities following multilevel laminectomy[2]. Since these original reports many others have detailed the problems with multilevel laminectomy. Yasuoka and associates reported in 1982 a follow-up study of 58 patients aged less than 25 years old who underwent multilevel laminectomy[30]. They found that spinal deformity developed in 46% of these patients less then 15 years of age and developed in all patients who had cervical laminectomies. Postoperative kyphosis has been reported by others to be as high as 50% in paediatric patients who undergo laminectomy for spinal cord tumour[16]. Mikawa and associates describe a group of older patients (mean age 50 years) who underwent multilevel cervical laminectomy[13]. They report that 36% showed postoperative changes in curvature type and 14% developed spinal deformities. Callahan[3] describes three groups of patients who have a higher probability of developing deformities: (1) patients aged less than 25 years, (2) patients who have had a laminectomy following trauma and in whom spinal stability is already compromised, (3) patients who have undergone laminectomy with extensive dissection of the facets.

Musculoligamentous insufficiency related to surgical stripping and denervation of the posterior paraspinal muscle complex has been suggested to be responsible for these progressive postlaminectomy deformities[20].

In an effort to reduce the rate of postlaminectomy complications, a number of innovative operative techniques have been developed[6, 7, 8, 9, 10, 12, 20, 21, 22, 25, 29]. All attempt to preserve some of the musculoligamentous attachments and bony posterior elements. Gros and associates describe their conservative lumbar laminectomy in which the laminectomy is performed after the spinous processes have been cut at their bases and retracted en bloc laterally[10]. Ohmori and associates recently described their "suspension laminotomy" in which they carefully preserve the posterior spinal ligaments, the paraspinal muscles and reestablish the posterior arch of the vertebra[20]. The technique of microdiscectomy was also developed to reduce the amount of tissue trauma necessary for the removal of herniated lumbar discs[1, 4, 6, 15, 26, 27, 28]. It was believed that by using the microscope and

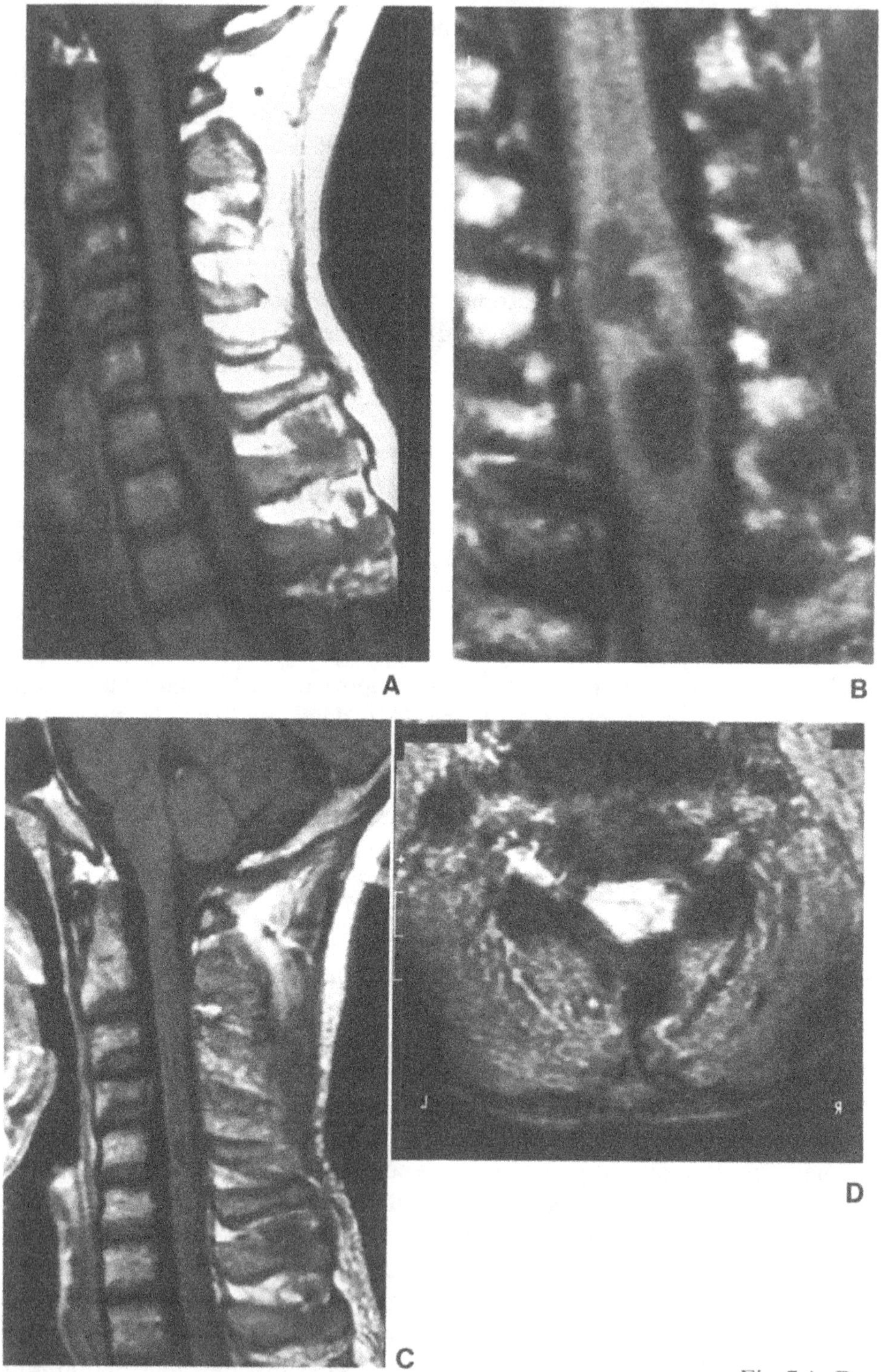

Fig. 7 A–D

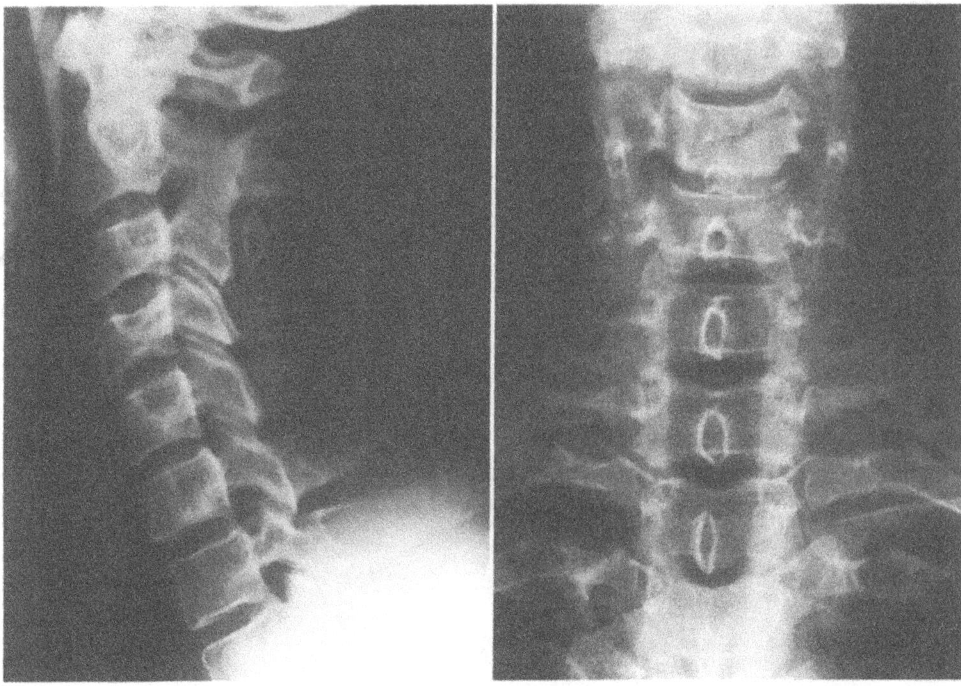

E F

Fig. 7. Case II: A 32 year old male orthopedic surgeon presented with a 4 week history of dysesthesias involving both arms. Physical examination revealed mild weakness of both arms, right worse than left. MRI revealed a cystic intramedullary tumour from C-4 to C-5 (A, B). The histologically confirmed ependymoma was removed through a C-3 to C-5 partial left hemilaminectomy. The patient's postoperative course was uneventful and he is working at full capacity as a surgeon without symptoms or neurologic deficits. An MRI done 6 months postoperatively demonstrates the tumour resection and normal spinal alignment (C, D). There was no postoperative vertebral column instability. Postoperative plain x-ray of cervical column and lateral view (E, F)

microsurgical technique, the disc could be removed with less dissection of the paravertebral muscles and ligamentum flavum resulting in less extradural scarring and less postoperative instability[27, 28].

In Zürich, the technique of hemilaminectomy is used routinely for the removal of all spinal cord tumours, with the exception of those extradural tumours which extensively invade local soft tissue structures bilaterally. With the aid of microneurosurgical techniques, the exposure provided by the hemilaminectomy is adequate for removal of intramedullary, intradural-extramedullary, and extradural tumours. The advantages of this technique versus the standard laminectomy are: (1) unilateral dissection of the paravertebral muscles and ligaments, and unilateral hemilaminar removal

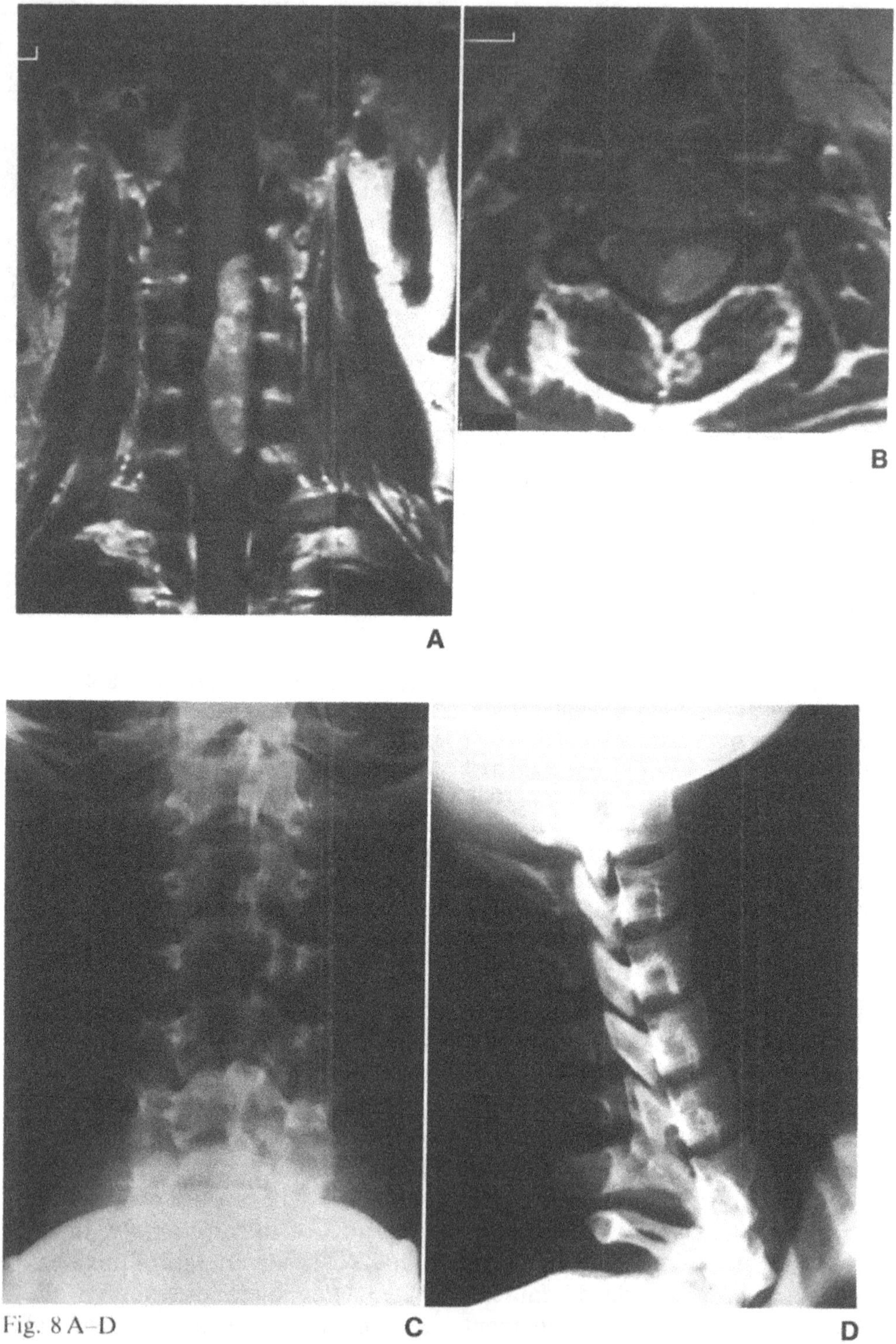

Fig. 8 A–D

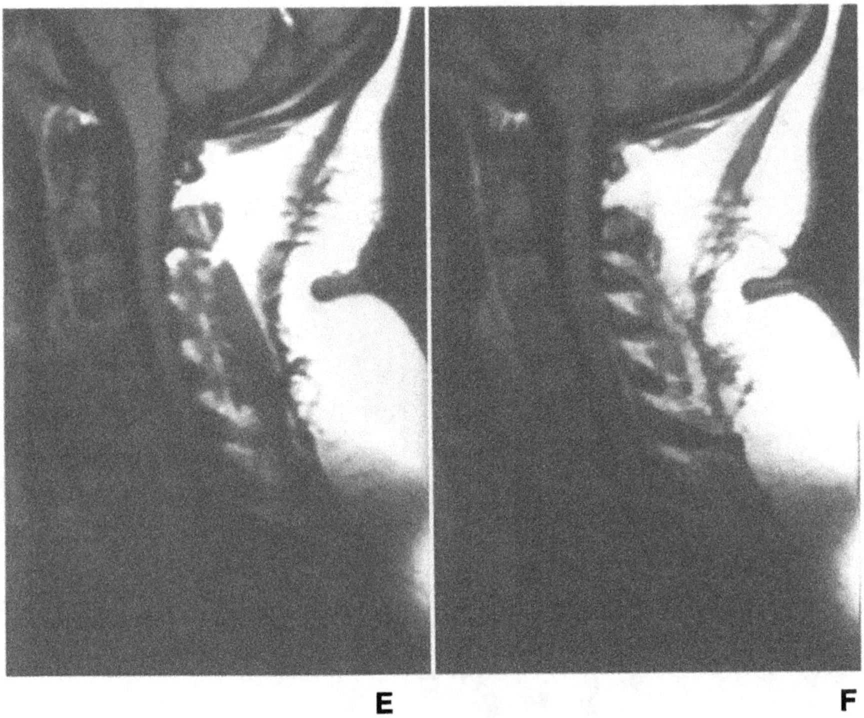

Fig. 8. Case III: A 15 year old girl presented with right leg weakness which recently developed after 2 years of right arm and shoulder weakness. MRI revealed a left sided intradural extramedullary tumour. 1 ½ × 5 cm at C-4 and C-5 (A, B). The tumour was resected through a partial left (C-4, C-5 and C-6) hemilaminectomy. Histology confirmed a neurinoma. Postoperatively, the patient made a rapid recovery and is symptom free without neurologic deficit. One year postoperatively plain x-ray and MRI demonstrate the tumour resection and hemilaminectomy with normal vertebral column alignment and stability (C, D, E, F)

provides a more stable spine postoperatively since the contralateral side remains intact; (2) the spinous process and intraspinal ligaments remain intact again providing more postoperative stability; (3) unilateral removal of the ligamentum flavum exposes less dural area thus less epidural scarring should occur postoperatively; and, (4) osseous protection for the spinal cord is improved since only a hemilaminectomy has been done.

In summary, by performing a hemilaminectomy and using microneurosurgical technique for the removal of almost all spinal cord tumours, the postoperative complications experienced following multilevel laminectomies can be much reduced. The extensive dissection of the multilevel laminectomy is eliminated and more of the natural protection for the spinal cord and biomechanical stability of the spine is preserved. The use of the

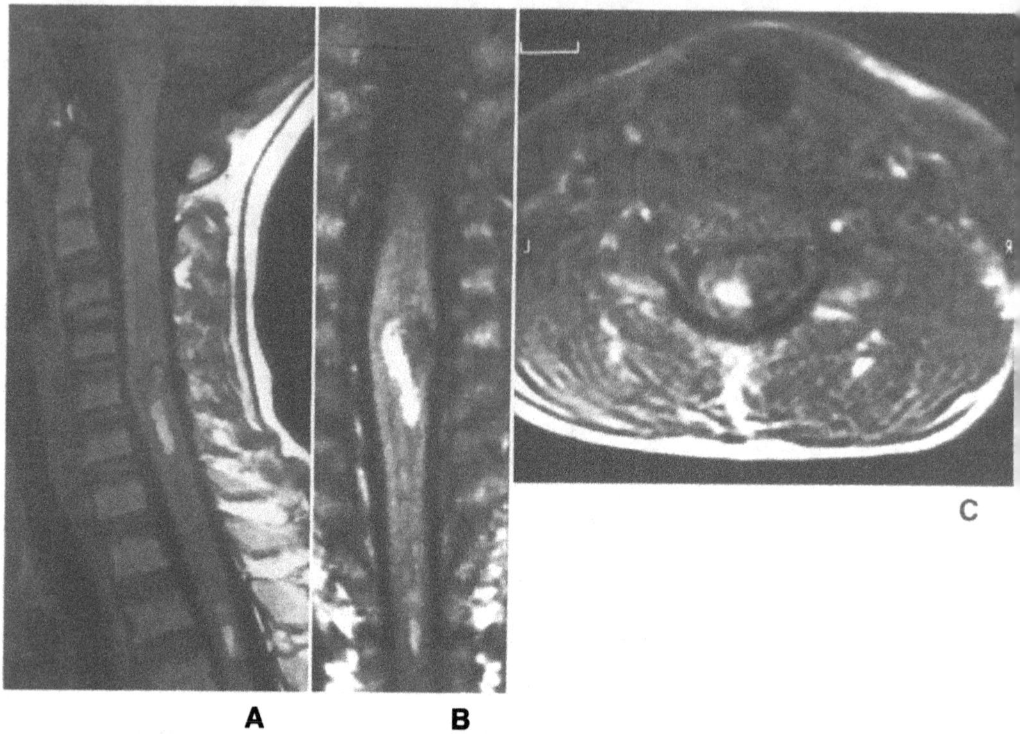

Fig. 9. Case IV: A 12 year old girl in July of 1988 developed an acute right sided arm weakness which rapidly progressed to a dense tetraparesis. She spontaneously improved over several hours but was left with a residual torticollis. The MRI was suggestive of an arteriovenous malformation at C-4, C-5 and C-6 (A, B, C). A selective spinal arteriogram confirmed an intramedullary AVM which was considered too risky for embolization (D, E, F, G). 3 weeks later a right partial (C-4, C-5 and C-6) hemilaminectomy was performed and the lesion removed. The patient had an uneventful recovery and is without symptoms or neurologic deficits. Postoperative MRI after 2 weeks demonstrated normal spinal alignment at the operative site (H, I). No instability of vertebral column

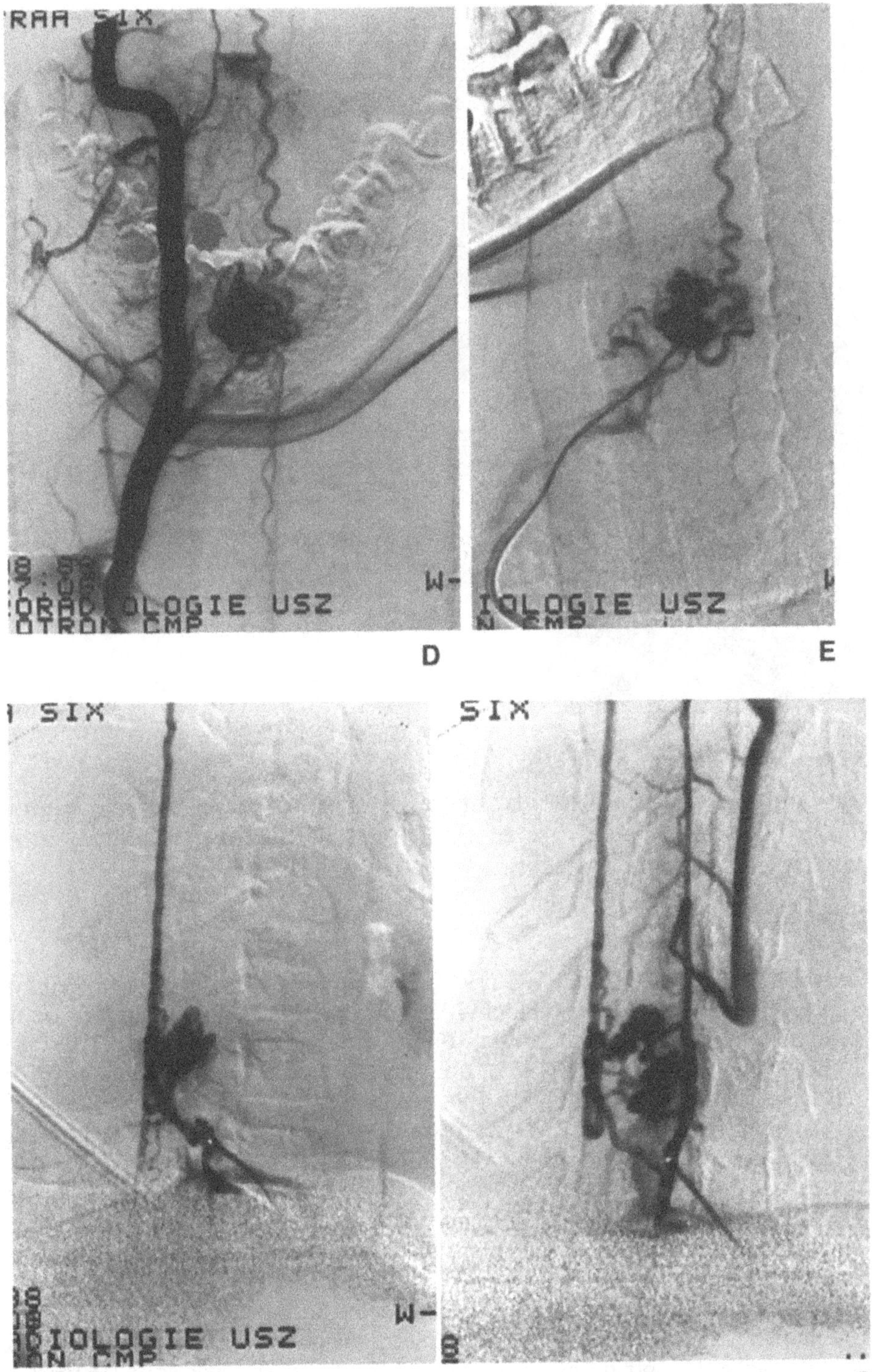

Fig. 9 D–G

H, I ►

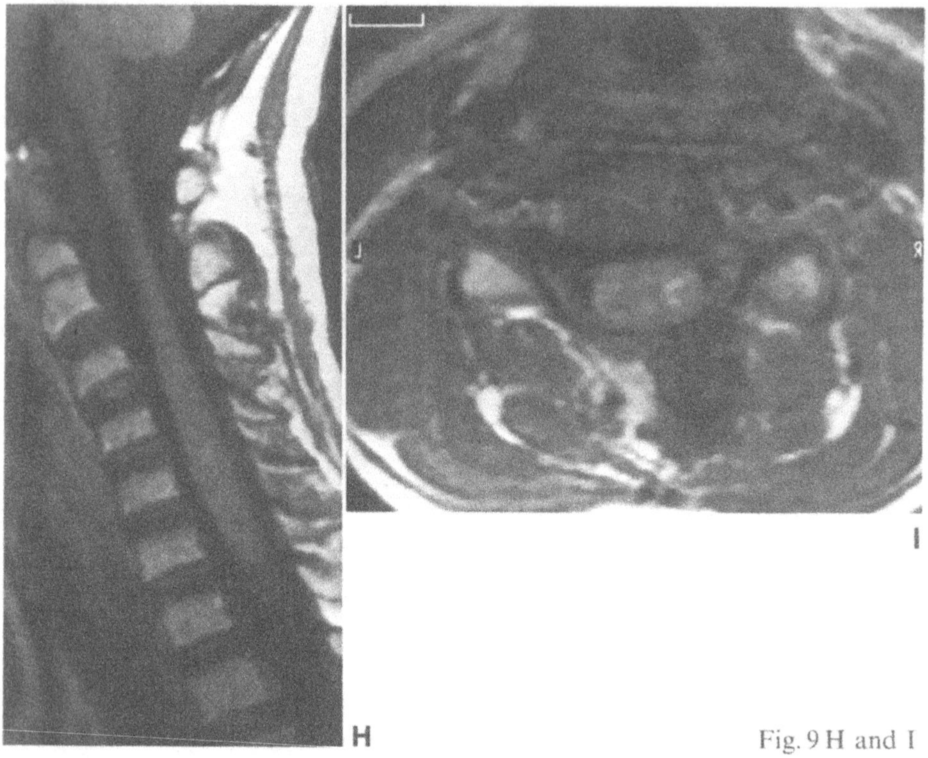

Fig. 9 H and I

hemilaminectomy has also advantages over other reconstructive laminotomies because it makes use of the spine's natural musculoligamentous stability and osseous protection.

References

1. Abernathey CD, Yaşargil MG (1990) Technique of microsurgery. In: Watkins RG, Williams RW, McCulloch JA, Young PH (eds) Microsurgery of the lumbar spine, Chapter 10, Aspen Publishers, Rockville, MD, pp 87–93
2. Bette H, Engelhardt H (1955) Folgezustände von Laminektomien an der Halswirbelsäule. Z Orthop 85: 564–573
3. Callahan RA, Johnson RM, Margolis RN *et al* (1977) Cervical facet fusion for control of instability following laminectomy. J Bone Joint Surg (Am) 59: 991–1002
4. Caspar W, Loew F (1977) Die mikrochirurgische Operation des lumbalen Bandscheibenvorfalls. Dtsch Aerztebl 13: 863–868
5. Cattell HS, Clark GL (1967) Cervical kyphosis and instability following multiple laminectomies in children. J Bone Joint Surg (Am) 49: 713–720
6. Chiou Sh-M, Eggert HR, Laborde G, Seeger W (1989) Microsurgical unilateral approaches for spinal tumour surgery: Eight years' experiences in 256 primary operated patients. Acta Neurochir (Wien) 100: 127–133

7. Eggert HR, Scheremet R, Seeger W, Gaitzsch J (1983) Unilateral microsurgical approaches to extramedullary spinal tumours: Operative technique and results. Acta Neurochir (Wien) 67: 245–253
8. Forni C, Regolo P (1986) Dolmen laminoplasty (Letter to the Editor). Spine 11: 853
9. Gilsbach J, Kaiser D, Eggert HR, Reif J (1985) Partielle Costotransversektomie und Thorakotomie in der Neurochirurgie. In: Hohmann D, Kügelgen B, Liebig K (eds) Neuroorthopädie 3. Springer, Berlin Heidelberg New York Tokyo, pp 219–225
10. Gros C, Frerebeau Ph, Privat JM *et al* (1983) Laminectomies conservatrices lombaires — Technique et resultats. Neurochirurgie 29: 207–209
11. Haft H, Ransohoff J, Carter S (1959) Spinal cord tumours in children. Pediatrics 23: 1152–1159
12. Hirabayashi K, Watanabe K, Wakano K *et al* (1983) Expansive open door laminoplasty for cervical spinal stenotic myelopathy. Spine 8: 693–699
13. Horsley V, Gowers WR (1888) A case of tumour of the spinal cord. Trans R Med Chir Soc Glasg 70: 377
14. Lee CK (1983) Lumbar spinal instability (olisthesis) after extensive posterior spinal decompression. Spine 8: 429–433
15. Loew F, Caspar W (1978) Surgical approach to lumbar disc herniations. In: Krayenbühl *et al* (eds) Advances and technical standards in neurosurgery, Vol 5. Springer, Wien New York, pp 153–174
16. Lonstein JE (1977) Post-laminectomy kyphosis. Clin Orthop 128: 93–100
17. Love JG (1966) Neurosurgical techniques: Laminectomy for removal of spinal cord tumour. J Neurosurg 25: 116–121
18. Markham JW (1951) Contribution of Alban G. Smith, of Kentucky, to the early history of surgery. J Ky Med Assoc 49: 398–401
19. Mikawa Y, Shikata J, Yamamuro T (1987) Spinal deformity and instability after multilevel cervical laminectomy. Spine 12: 6–11
20. Ohmori I, Ishida Y, Suzuki K (1987) Suspension laminotomy; a new surgical technique for compression myelopathy. Neurosurgery 21:950–957
21. Raimondi AJ, Gutierrez FA (1979) Reconstruction of the posterior vertebral arch and laminotomy for intraspinal surgery. In: Ransohoff J (ed) Modern technics in surgery-neurosurgery, Futura Publishing Co, vol 10. Mt Kisco, New York, pp 1–7
22. Seeger W (1982) Microsurgery of the spinal cord and surrounding structures: Anatomical and technical principles. Springer, Wien New York
23. Sim FH, Svien HJ, Bickell WH (1974) Swan-Neck deformity following extensive cervical laminectomy. J Bone Joint Surg 56A: 564–580
24. Tachdjian MO, Matson DO (1965) Orthopedic aspects of intraspinal tumours in infants and children. J Bone Joint Surg (Am) 47:223–248
25. Tsuji H (1982) Laminoplasty for patients with compressive myelopathy due to so-called spinal canal stenosis in cervical and thoracic regions. Spine 7: 28–34
26. Watkins RG, Williams RW, McCulloch JA, Young PH (1990) Microsurgery of the lumbar spine. Aspen Publishers, Rockville, Maryland, 271 pp

27. Williams RW (1978) Microlumbar discectomy: A conservative surgical approach to the virgin herniated disc. Spine 3: 175–182
28. Yaşargil MG (1977) Microsurgical operation for herniated lumbar disc. In: Advances in neurosurgery, Vol 4. Springer, Berlin Heidelberg New York, p 81
29. Yaşargil MG, Perneczky A (1976) Operative Behandlung der intramedullären spinalen Tumoren. In: Schiefer W, Wieck HH (eds) Spinale raumfordernde Prozesse. Verlag Peri Med, Erlangen, pp 299–312
30. Yasuoka S, Peterson HA, MacCarty CS (1982) Incidence of spinal column deformity after multilevel laminectomy in children and adults. J Neurosurg 57: 441–445

Organization of the Primary Transportation of Head Injuries and Other Emergencies in the Federal Republic of Germany*

H. Dietz

Neurochirurgische Klinik, Medizinische Hochschule Hannover, (Federal Republic of Germany)

With 2 Figures

From ancient times until recently First Aid has been rendered to the injured by laymen. Organized medical assistance was not available. It was Larrey, Napoleon's Chief Surgeon, who in 1792 first introduced military medical emergency care. Army surgeons were stationed close to the front line in readiness for the expected casualty, who were brought to them in horse drawn wagons. It meant that 48 hrs. passed before the wounded received surgical attention; 46% of them died.

The problems of modern primary surgical attention were, in the main, organizational: in as much as it concerned the reduction of the so-called "care-free interval". This interval refers to the inevitable time-lapse experienced by the wounded before receiving medical attention. This period amounted to 12 to 24 hours in the 1st world war with a 8.5% loss of life. Better organization in the 2nd world war contracted this time down to 6–12 hrs. with a subsequent reduction in the loss of life to 5.8%. Nevertheless the time-interval for the evacuation of head injuries continued to average 24 hrs. The reasons for this were twofold: firstly these casualties required evacuation to specialist units and secondly closed head injuries were not so readily diagnosed as injuries to the trunk and limbs. During the conflict in Vietnam the Americans used helicopters for the immediate evacuation of the wounded. This achieved a reduction of the care-free interval to 65 minutes on average, and a figure of 1.7% regarding loss of life.

Already in 1938 Kirschner in Germany raised the question of the demand for the doctor to come to injured persons rather than vice versa.

---

* FRG means West Germany and West-Berlin before the unification of Germany on October 3, 1990.

Yet it was only in 1957 through the initiative of the surgeon K. H. Bauer that the use of the "flying squad" became a reality. Since then rapid development of the Emergency Services has been seen, not only in Germany but also in other countries of Europe, especially in England progress was fast, as the example of Rowbotham's organizational plans show.

In the Federal Republic of Germany further development led to the introduction of helicopter evacuation. In 1971 helicopter "Christoph 1" was first used in Munich and in 1972 three further helicopters "Christoph 2, 3 and 4" were stationed in Frankfurt/Main, Cologne and Hannover respectively. So today a system of air-evacuation exists, using over 36 helicopter bases covering the whole of the country as shown in Fig. 1. The whole of the Emergency Services of the Federal Republic of Germany are by law part of the State's Health Services, jointly financed by the Federal Ministries of the Interior and of Defence. The organization of the Emergency Service itself is the task of the regions but the District General Hospital and its catchment area is responsible for its ambulance and helicopter headquarters including the provision of emergency medical cover. Such cover is almost entirely provided by hospital doctors, particularly experienced in Intensive Care, Anaesthesia and Emergency Surgery.

Of importance for the further shortening of the care-free interval is the mode of transport. Five different types of transport vehicles are available in the Federal Republic of Germany:

1. Ambulance Type I ("Krankentransportwagen"): This vehicle is used for the movement of non-urgent patients. It is equipped for simple First Aid.

2. Ambulance Type II ("Rettungswagen"): This is a much bigger vehicle supplied with a comprehensive range of medical equipment as laid down by international agreement. It is manned by two ambulance men, but not a doctor.

3. Ambulance Type III ("Notarztwagen"): This is a vehicle for the Emergency Medical Team of the Flying Squad. The vehicle is stationed at the hospital and affords a higher quality of rescue. Two patients can be cared for and the compliment of 4 staff consists of a driver, two ambulance men and one casualty surgeon. The squad is available 24 hrs. round the clock. The staffing ratio is relatively high, requiring 10 ambulance men and 4 doctors.

4. Ambulance Type IV ("Notarzteinsatzfahrzeug"): We refer to this type of vehicle as the "emergency call in". This machine is equipped with all important medical instruments and drugs. The use of this ambulance is cheaper than Type III and is manned by one ambulance man and one doctor. Over the 24 hrs. it represents a considerable saving in personnel compared with the Type III ambulance.

This ambulance, Type IV, works on the so-called rendezvous-system as follows: as medical demand at an accident may require besides this Ambulance, Type IV, additional help, Ambulance Type II is also dispatched; if according to the need of the injured a medical escort to the hospital is necessary, the doctor of the Type IV Ambulance accompanies the injured in the Type II Ambulance for practical purposes converting it into a flying squad ambulance as described under Type III. Should no medical escort be required, then this ambulance, Type IV is ready for the next call and the simultaneously dispatched Ambulance Type II evacuates the casualty in company of the two ambulance men to the hospital.

5. The most expensive method of transportation is by *Helicopter Air Ambulance* ("Rettungshubschrauber"). Among the advantages are a greater catchment area, speed up to 200 km/hour, not dependent upon road conditions or traffic density. The injured can be flown directly to the specialty unit with less movement and disturbance during the transfer, an important consideration where spinal and head injuries are concerned. One drawback of helicopter evacuation is its dependence upon daylight and the weather as it flies by ground landmarks, and so cannot be used in darkness or in snow or fog. Per year these adverse conditions prevented in Germany the use of helicopter on 3 to 10 days (6 days on average in Hannover). A further drawback of the older helicopters (Type MBB BO 105) is the cramped space available which severely restricts what can be done for the patient during the flight. The newer types (MBB K 117) are much better in this respect since there is more room.

An *Ambulance Headquarters* coordinates and decides upon previously agreed criteria what method of evacuation is appropriate and what type of ambulance is sent to the site of an accident. If the Flying Squad is part of the team the Casualty Surgeon will decide on the spot:

1. priorities of medical treatment,
2. whether more medical or technical equipment is needed,
3. to which hospital the injured will be sent.

The Casualty Surgeon will know the hospitals of the area, he may have to overrule local Emergency Services, and will therefore be of consultant status in Emergency Surgery and Intensive Care. He will be able to carry our endotracheal intubation, institute positive pressure respiration, pleural drainage, dress an open head-injury, decide upon urgent medication and the type and amount of immediate intravenous transfusion.

The year 1985 will be taken as an example to illustrate the method and use of these various types of ambulance. In the Federal Republic of Germany 560 000 emergency calls were answered in 1985: 47% constituted medical emergencies, 15.7% traffic accidents, the remainder, 37.3%, included accidents at work, sport and leisure. 54.9% were dealt with by

Ambulances of Type III described above, 40.7% by Ambulances of Type IV and 4.4% by Helicopter Air Ambulances Type V.

The reason for the use of a helicopter is given in a review of 248.000 emergency calls: 42% in traffic accidents, 23% in medical emergencies, 10% in accidents at work, 8% for miscellaneous reasons and in 17% for secondary transports, which means transfer from the primary hospital to another hospital with possibilities for specialist treatment, say a Regional Neurosurgical Centre.

The mode of calling the emergency surgeon, the time it takes for him to reach the scene of the accident, the method of transfer of the injured to the hospital, all in all the effectiveness of the primary care possibilities, will be illustrated by taking the catchment area of the Hannover Medical School as an example. It is to be emphasized that the Institution has a central Accident and Emergency facility capable of dealing with every type of urgent case, not only accidents. The Medical School has at its disposal its own Helicopter Air Ambulance, one Type III Ambulance and one Type IV Ambulance, each with its own personnel on emergency stand-by 24 hours a day. In addition to this commitment Hannover deals with referals from the adjoining catchment areas 13, 19, and 30 (Fig. 1), each served by its own helicopter.

In the first 13 years of existence of a helicopter and other types of ambulances in Hannover, 30.084 emergency calls habe been registered. Of these 14.694 cases came by helicopter and 15.390 by other types of ambulances. Taking into account the area of operation (radius 30–50 km for the helicopter and 6–8 km for the ambulance and the time taken to reach the scene of the accident (helicopter 5–25 minutes, ambulances 5–15 minutes), we were able to establish that within 10 minutes the ambulance was on the spot in 22% of all cases and the helicopter in 65%.

This immediate and fast availability has on average reduced the care-free interval to 10 minutes and the time taken from the arrival of the doctor at the patient's side until his admission to our Emergency and Casualty Department to 30 minutes.

Of these approx. 30.000 emergency admissions during the first 13 years, 23% arrived in coma, 57% had head-injuries (alone or together with other lesions), 40% fractures of the extremities, 24% chest injuries and 30% had breathing difficulties.

Irrespective of the mode of answering the emergency call and with what type of transport the emergencies reached the hospital, it was established during the last few years that approx. 20.000 patients of this category per annum were admitted to our Institution. About half these cases (10.000) had head-injuries either alone or associated with other trauma and 10% (approx. 2.000 head-injuries per year), required neurosurgical attention, irrespective of other surgical needs. Approx. 10% needed neurosurgical operation (in 1986, for example, there were 180 such cases and 210 in 1988). A further 200 cases were admitted without operation to the neurosurgical intensive care unit because of traumatic cerebral oedema and coma and the need for active ventilatory support.

About half of these 20.000 annual trauma cases had sustained multiple injuries, not only involving the limbs but also the trunk, thorax, vertebral column and head. In severe cases specialist teams will decide the priority of treatment. The most urgent need for diagnosis and treatment will be determined as far as possible taking into account the primary condition. In rare instances two specialist teams may operate simultaneously, as for instance for extradural haematoma and abdominal or thoracic trauma. However, this occurs only 2 to 3 times a year in our experience.

Difficulties arise not infrequently with primary diagnostic procedures, such as computertomography or angiography, since these facilities are not situated in the immediate vicinity of the Casualty Department. The patient will have to be moved to the X-ray department, perhaps some 200 m.Though other supportive treatment continues in the meantime, it is still possible that the time taken for these diagnostic procedures may be 30 to 60 minutes. As previously mentioned, what might be termed the preclinical phase, namely the time elapsing from the doctor arriving at the scene of the accident to the patients' arrival at the hospital, averages out at 30 minutes. This period is therefore exceeded by the time required for establishing a definitive diagnosis, confirmed radiologically.

In principle all patients with head injury or a suspicion there of on initial diagnosis are submitted to computertomography. Depending on the clinical condition in cases with cerebral oedema and not absolutely clear cut minor contusional haemorrhages the computertomography is repeated within 2–8 hours in order to exclude any developing focal surgical space-occupying haemorrhage.

One must not overlook the fact that the reduction of the preclinical phase to about 30 minutes by the use of modern methods outlined above, has brought about new problems: the rapid delivery of the most seriously injured cases to the Casualty Department irrespective of their chances of survival has not only raised the demand for greater medical and nursing care but also inevitably the average mortality figures of Intensive Care Units.

The emergency doctor in transit whether by ambulance or helicopter to our Medical School Hospital requests the presence of the various specialists on arrival according to his assessment of his patients' injuries; Ophthalmology for obvious eye-trauma, ENT for bleeding from the ear, nose or throat, colleagues from General-, Abdominal- or Chest-Surgery for clear abdominal and thoracic injuries and not least the neurosurgeon on call. It has to be admitted that a consequence of the presence in the

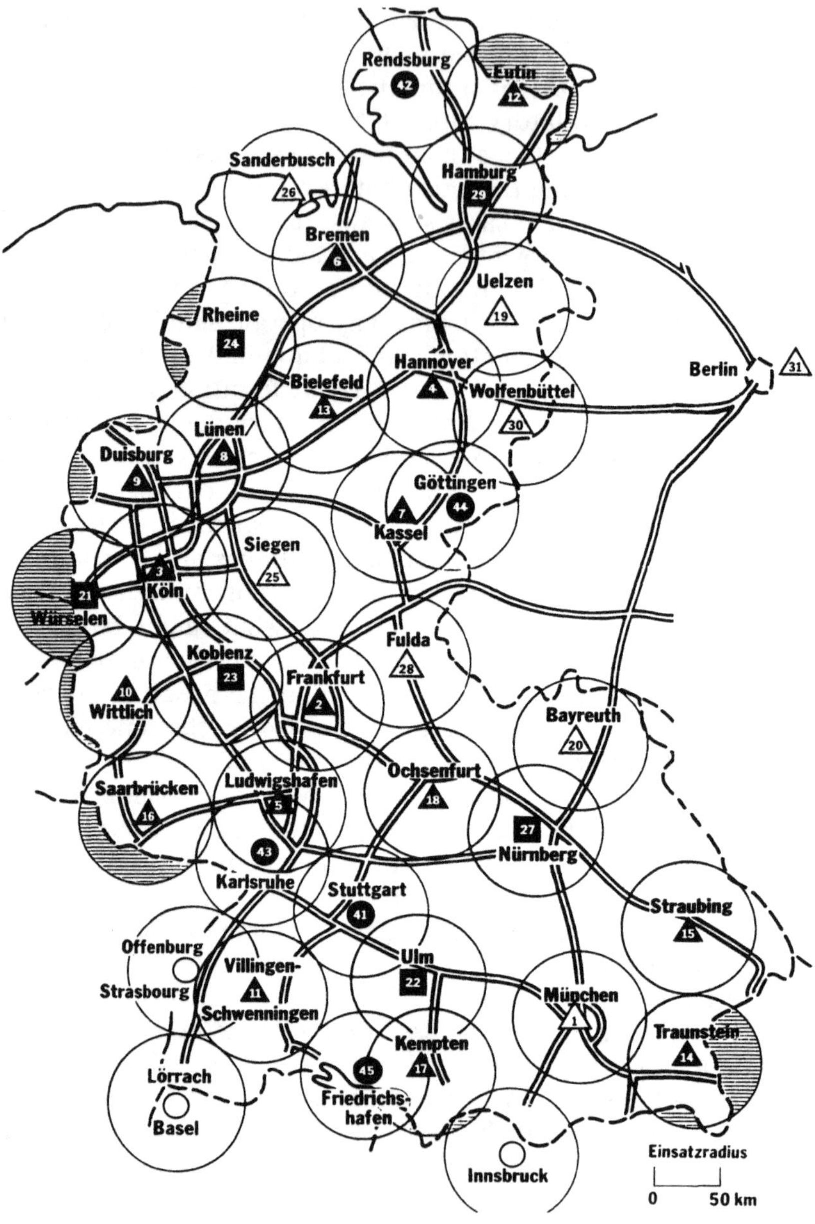

Fig. 1. Basis of air-evacuation

Casualty Department of several doctors from the various disciplines alerted, creates a crowd around the seriously injured patient or patients, particularly those with multiple trauma, and can prevent the orderly medical care required especially when opinions differ regarding priorities of treatment.

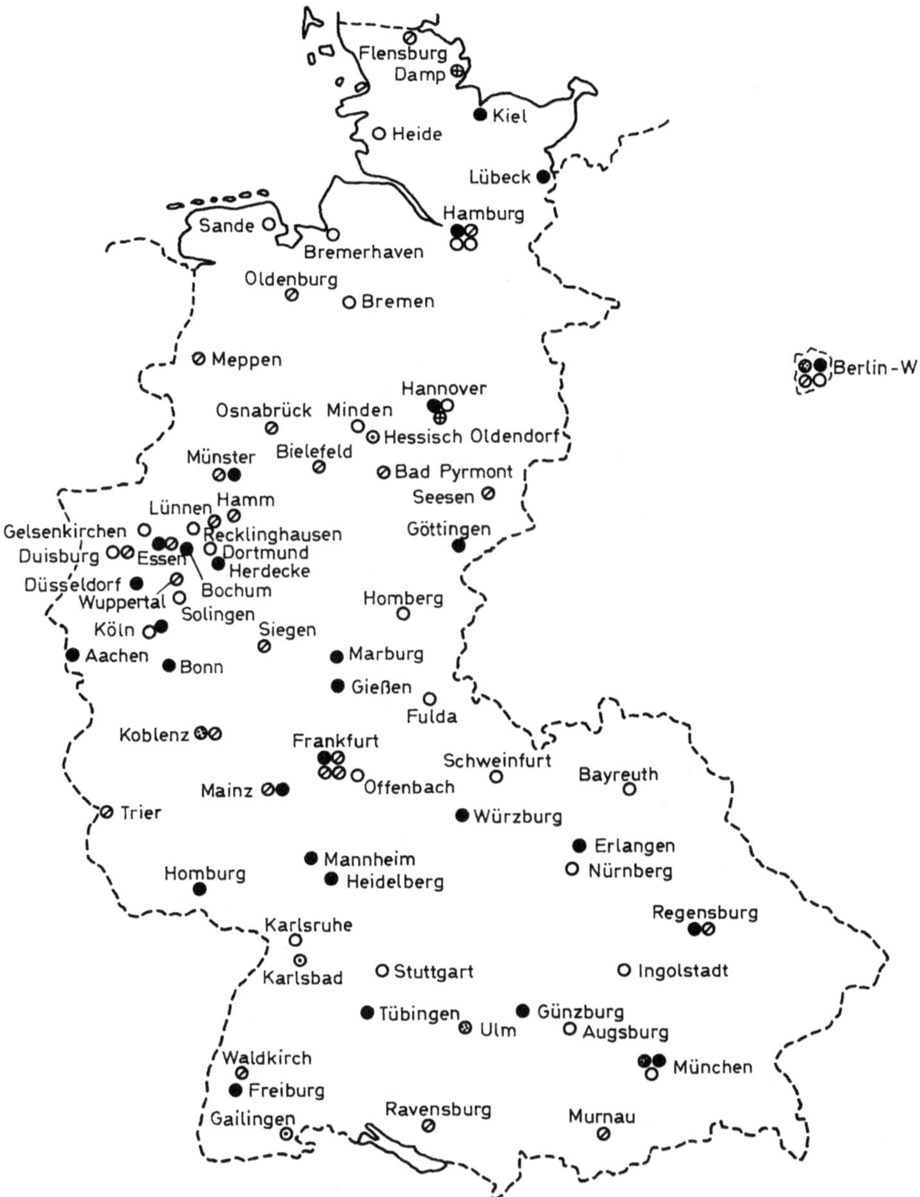

Fig. 2. Neurosurgical Units in the Federal Republic of Germany

Furthermore the performance of several examinations by specialists can prolong the time before a diagnosis is reached and engender a delay for urgent preoperative investigations, such as computertomography or angiography.

Unfortunately right from the start our situation is such in Hannover, that we had to accept a considerable distance between the Casualty and Emergency and the Radiology or Neuroradiology Department. The intubated patient on a ventilator has to be transported within the hospital, he may have to be moved into various positions, a risk for the seriously injured patient which has to be accepted. Many personnel will be tied up, much valuable time can be lost, leading to delay in performing a possibly urgent operation.

We have found that in order to overcome these difficulties it is important always to have available two fully-trained senior doctors of consultant status accredited to the Emergency and Casualty Department. Their duty is to be responsible for the care of these patients and it will be within their competence to decide which specialty will take priority in that care.

It is, however, important to determine that this system of medical care is of clear advantage for the patient.

As of December 1989 there were 83 independent Neurosurgical Units in the Federal Republic of Germany including West-Berlin with approx. 5.000 beds (Fig. 2). More than half of these have their own Intensive Care Units, while the remainder participate in the General Intensive Care Unit of their hospital, run by Anaesthesiologists.

Comparison of Fig. 1 with Fig. 2 will show that a neurosurgical emergency air evacuation by helicopter will be rapid to the appropriate centre, where specialist care will be equally rapidly available. It is likely that the staffing complement of some units is not always optimal and that the example, proved over the years in Hannover, of such cooperation between the specialties and the methods of evacuation to the hospital cannot always be achieved. However, it is always possible to transfer a particularly difficult case from the primary hospital, where treatment was initiated, to a Neurosurgical University Clinic or large District General Hospital with a full complement of neurosurgical staff and facilities, when total care can be provided and completed.

The reduction of time of the care-free interval (time from injury to start of treatment) has been described as we have achieved it at the Medical School Hannover, making the best use of all means and methods of rescue for the patient. It is to be emphasized that the evolution to the present structure of organization over many years was only possible through the hard work, great devotion and much good will of all parties concerned. Only the willing cooperation of all has over the last two decades allowed us to reach this standard in Hannover; it was not only done by rules and regulations. It has been a particular pleasure to note during this period how the satisfaction of working together in constant readiness has built up the ideal of all for all in the service of the patient.

References

1. Arntz H-R, Storch WH, Völler H, Goecke J, Schröder R (1990) Ein Jahr Rettungshubschrauber in Berlin (West). Der Notarzt 6: 1–4
2. Börner M, Soldner E (1986) Statistische Auswertung der Einsätze der 3 Notarztwagen im Rettungsdienst der Stadt Frankfurt vom 8.6.1966 bis 31.12.1984. Der Notarzt 2: 73–78
3. Contzen H (1986) Notfall- und Rettungswesen. In: Probst J (Hrsg) Unfallheilkunde 1986: 69–73 Demeter-Verlag, Gräfelfing
4. Dietz H: Organisatorische Probleme der Erstversorgung der Schädelhirnverletzten. Unfall-Symposium Pörtschach (Kärnten) 25.–27.09.1987
5. Engelhardt GH (1985) Schädel-Hirn-Trauma: Versorgung am Unfallort. Rettungsdienst, Heft 2, 73–77
6. Karimi-Nejad A (1985) Diagnostische Strategie und Akutversorgung beim Schädel-Hirn-Trauma. Diagnostik und Intensivmedizin 10: 8–17
7. Kirschner M (1938) Der Verkehrsunfall und seine Behandlung. Arch Klin Chir 193: 230–257
8. Kugler E (1986) Grundlagen der Luftrettung in der Bundesrepublik Deutschland. Der Notarzt 2: 147–149
9. Otte D (1968) Verkehrsunfallforschung. In: Probst J (Hrsg) Unfallheilkunde 1968: 65–68 Demeter-Verlag, Gräfelfing
10. Richard KE (1985) Neurochirurgische Aspekte in der klinischen Erstversorgung. Anästh Intensivmedizin 26: 199–205
11. Rowbotham GF (1968) Acute injuries of the head, 4th Ed. E & S Livingstone, Edinburgh London
12. Soldner E, Börner M (1986) Statistische Auswertung der Einsätze des Rettungshubschraubers Christoph II über einen Zeitraum von 10 Jahren. Der Notarzt 2: 79–82
13. Tönnis W *et al* (1968) Organisation der Behandlung schwerer Schädel-Hirn-Verletzungen. In: Arbeit und Gesundheit, Heft 79. Thieme, Stuttgart

Advances in Drug Delivery Systems and Applications in Neurosurgery

Y. LAZORTHES, B. SALLERIN-CAUTE, J. C. VERDIE, and R. BASTIDE

University Neurosurgical Clinic, Medical Faculty of Rangueil, Université Paul Sabatier, Toulouse (France)

With 5 Figures

Contents

The principle of direct administration of repeated doses of drugs either at or close to their site of action in the central nervous system is based on:

– the identification of specific receptors and neuro-active endogenous peptides which has considerably advanced our understanding of the functioning of the central nervous system. The notion of chemical transmission of information in specific pathways now underlies the early electrical model of Galvani.

– better understanding of the pharmacological action of endogenous and exogenous ligands, which was led to the development of specific and highly active drugs. Such drugs are now employed routinely in the treatment of chronic conditions such as intractable pain or spasticity. In the near future, it may also be possible to treat other neurological diseases by manipulation of the specific neuromediators or neuromodulators involved.

– the fact that high doses of drug are often required via the systemic route, giving rise to adverse reactions in other parts of the organism before the active agent reaches the target organ. Many drugs do not readily cross the blood-brain barrier, and are degraded in the periphery either in the digestive tract, liver or kidneys. This means that the therapeutic ratio is low for many drugs. Moreover, distribution in the central nervous system itself is not localized to the site of action (spinal cord for example) which can give rise to supra-spinal side effects.

– advances in technology which have stimulated development of implantable systems enabling local or regional administration of many drugs employed in endocrinology, oncology and neurology.

In neurology, treatment of chronic cancer pain using an implanted system for the intrathecal and intraventricular injection of morphine was first described in 1978. This technique is now in routine use. Over the past 6 years, severe spasticity of central origin has also been treated effectively by intrathecal administration of Baclofen.

We will discuss these two applications (pain and spasticity) which are now a routine part of conservative neurosurgery. We will also mention other indications for "pharmacological neurosurgery" which are currently being tested for effectiveness and safety.

1. Implantable Drug Delivery Systems

The main objectives of drug delivery systems (DDS) are to:

a) provide a non-invasive access to the various compartments of the central nervous system (epidural space, lumbar sub-arachnoid space, cisterns, ventricles, parenchyma, etc). or vascular system,

b) enable single or repeated administration of drugs or contrast media,

c) obtain samples of CSF or blood,

d) prevent leakage of active principle to other organs,

e) employ drugs which are not degraded in contact with the generally inert biocompatible materials used in the construction of the delivery systems,

f) enable treatment on a out-patient basis without risk to the patient.

DDS are implanted subcutaneously, and are connected to flexible catheters whose distal end is placed in the zone or site of action. Various systems from single access ports to micropumps are now available for administration of repeated bolus doses, or continuous or programmable infusions.

1.1 Access Ports

These are small volume rigid chambers placed in contact with the compartment to be infused. They are designed to replace lumbar or intraventricular puncture or intravascular injection by a simple subcutaneous injection. The first systems which were used for intra-ventricular injections consisted of a dome-shaped silicone capsule derived from an Ommaya reservoir. They were then modified by moving the catheter junction to the periphery. The Unidose reservoir developed by Cordis* is one of the most widely used. It is available in two sizes (1 and 2 ml). It has a stainless steel base-plate which prevents the injection needle passing right through it. However, its dome shape and its thin wall means that it is not self-sealing, and it can only be used a few times, even with fine needles (25 G), before it starts to leak. It is thus not used for repeated chronic administration.

Pharmacia have developed improved access ports under the trade name Port-A-Cath®. They are constructed of stainless steel or titanium closed by a membrane or self-sealing compressed silicone stopper (septum). This septum has a diameter of 10 mm with a surface area around 1 cm^2 and a thickness of 5 to 6 mm. The depth of the chamber under the membrane is between 5 and 8 mm giving a total capacity of 0.5 ml. Over 1000 punctures and injections ats can be made without leakage using a 22 G needle with a Huber type point.

The access port is joined by a safety connector and an anti-kinking system to the catheter whose diameter depends on the actual site of infusion. The Port-A-Cath® system is now widely used in oncology. Various manufacturers now produce similar systems using other biocompatible materials such as stainless steel, polysulfone, reinforced silicone, etc, and more than 20 different models are now available. Examples are the Life-Port®, Infuse-Port®, Polysit®.

The MPAP® system developed by Cordis is of interest as it is equipped with a 7 to 8 mm thick septum with a larger surface area (2.7 cm^2) than

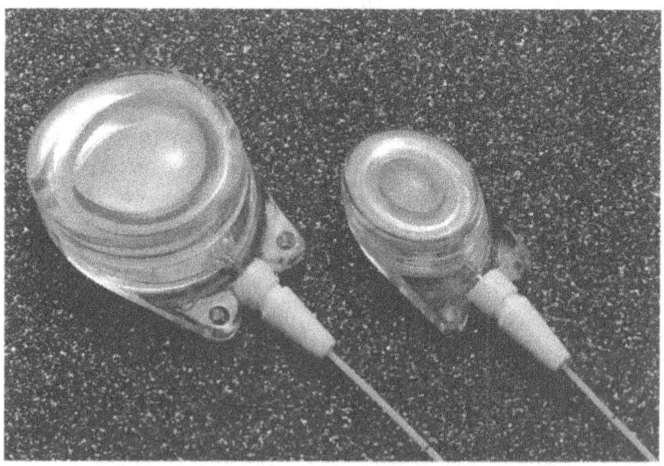

Fig. 1. Cordis Multipurpose Access Port (MPAP)tm and Miniporttm for intrathecal or vascular access

* Cordis Biot Operation, Route des Dolines, Sophia-Antipolis, 06560 Valbonne, France.

the other systems. It is thus easily located under the skin, and can be implanted at an oblique angle to facilitate insertion of indwelling needles for infusion via a portable miniature pump. A miniature version, the Miniport®, with an oblique silicone septum (0.6 cm^2, 6 mm thick) with a 5 to 8 mm deep reservoir is also available. It is employed for intra-arterial administration of drugs used in chemotherapy, and also for intrathecal administration in children as well as adults (Fig. 1).

These systems have the advantage of ease of use and low cost, although the need for repeated injections (daily or even several times a day) into the reservoir restricts the patients mobility, and increases the risk of infection.

1.2 Implantable Pumps

These DDS have reservoirs of varying capacities (generally 12–50 ml) which can be refilled by injection through a self-sealing septum. The freedom of movement of the patient will clearly be influenced by size of the reservoir. The safety and reliability depend in the accuracy and adaptability of the infusion rate (pulsatile or continuous). The different systems can be classified in terms of their programmability, from simple pulsatile pumps to fully programmable, remote-controlled electric pumps.

1.2.1 Pulsatile Pumps

These are purely mechanical hand-operated systems. The Secor® pump produced by Cordis consists of three one-way valves in series which delivers constant volume boluses (0.1 ml ± 10%) (Fig. 2). The dosage is adjusted by varying the number of boluses and/or the concentration of the active principle.

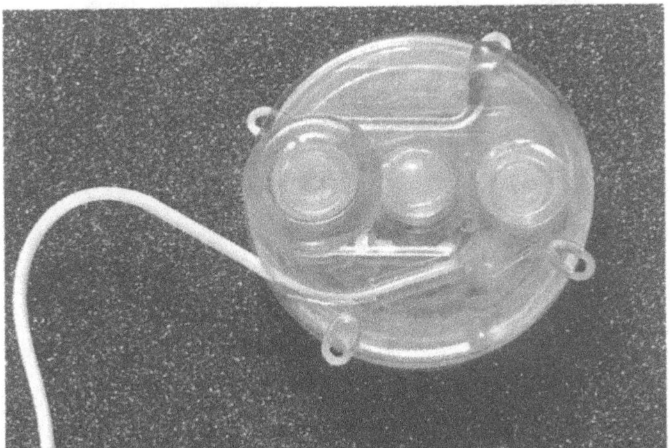

Fig. 2. Cordis Secor^tm implantable multidose reservoir

The body of the pump is made of polysulfone (6 cm diam, 1.4 cm deep) and it only weights 45 grams. The useable capacity of the flexible Teflon reservoir attached to the bottom of the unit is 12 to 15 ml.On the first generation of Secor pumps, the two push buttons could not be located easily under the skin. The pump was primed by pressing one button and drug was injected by pressing the other one. The two buttons on the second generation now protrude slightly more, and they incorporate a tactile feedback with a click so that the operator knows that the pump has been operated effectively, and the dose administered.

Although the relative inaccuracy of the Secor pump restricts its application especially for administration of drugs such as Baclofen, its safety and low cost make it particularly suitable for intrathecal administration of opiates in the treatment of intractable cancer pain.

1.2.2 Continuous Flow Pumps

An example is the Infusaid* (model 400) first produced in 1969. The drug solution is forced through the system by a gas (Freon) contained in an external chamber connected to the reservoir containing the drug via flexible bellows made of titanium. At a given temperature, the liquid phase of Freon is in equilibrium with the gas phase and exerts a constant pressure (450 mmHg at 37 °C) thus expelling the drug solution progressively through a regulator valve and bacterial filter (0.22 microns) into the catheter. Re-

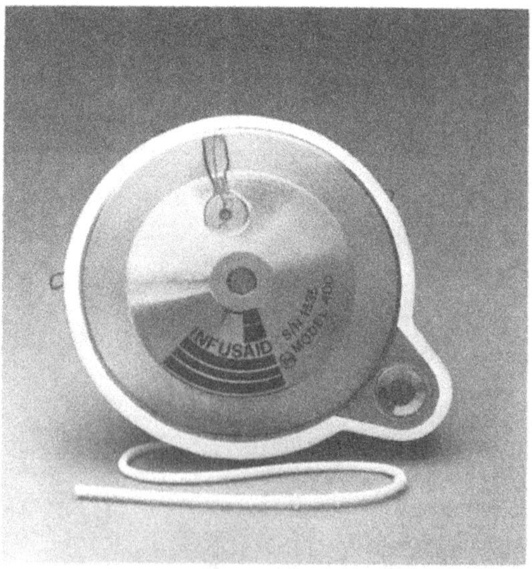

Fig. 3. Infusaid Model 400 continuous flow pump

* Infusaid Inc., 1400 Providence Highway, Norwood, MA 02062, U.S.A.

filling the pump expands the bellows and compresses the propellant gas to a liquid, thereby reactivating the pump.

Inert materials such as titanium, polypropylene, stainless steel, silicone and Teflon are used in the parts of the pump that come in contact with the drug. It has an empty weight of 208 grams with a reservoir capacity of 47 ml, and is the largest currently available. Model 400 (Fig. 3) is also equipped with a side-port enabling administration of more than one drug and verification of the permeability of the catheter. The flow rates of the pumps are factory-set to between 1.0 and 6.0 ml/24 h, and this flow rate cannot be altered after implantation. The only way of altering the dose is by changing the drug concentration in the reservoir. A further disadvantage is that the flow rate depends of the temperature of the patient and the atmospheric pressure. Furthermore, in emergency, the infusion can only be stopped by draining the reservoir. These disadvantages restrict the use of these DDS in neurosurgery when powerful centrally acting drugs are employed, especially if there are no antagonists available, as is the case for Baclofen. On the other hand, these pumps are well suited for intrathecal or intravenous infusion of the relatively large amounts of drugs used in chemotherapy where accurate dosage is not usually required. The new generation of continuous-flow Infusaid pumps are now fitted with flow regulators.

In 1989, Therex* introduced an implantable constant-flow pump with 30 ml capacity employing the same principle as the Infusaid 400 system. There is a yet insufficient experience with this system to come to any firm conclusions, but it is likely to have the same advantages and disadvantages of the Infusaid 400 system.

1.2.3 Programmable Pumps

These are generally electromechanical pumps of the peristaltic type powered by a lithium battery. Their built-in electronics can be remotely controlled from an external programming unit. The most sophisticated and most widely employed in neurosurgery is the Synchromed system manufactured by Medtronic**. The titanium and silicone unit (70 mm diameter, 27.5 mm deep) has an empty weight of 185 grams (Fig. 4) and a useable capacity of 18.0 ml with a 2.4 ml dead space. Energy is provided by a lithium thionyl chloride battery with an average life of 3 years at a flow rate of 1.5 ml/24 h.

The infusion parameters can be remotely controlled, and the flow rate can be adjusted over a range of 0.004 ml/h to 0.9 ml/h. The accuracy of

---

* Therex Corp., 1600 Providence Highway, Walpole, MA 02081, U.S.A.

** Medtronic Inc., 7000 Central Av. NE, Minneapolis, MN 55432, U.S.A.

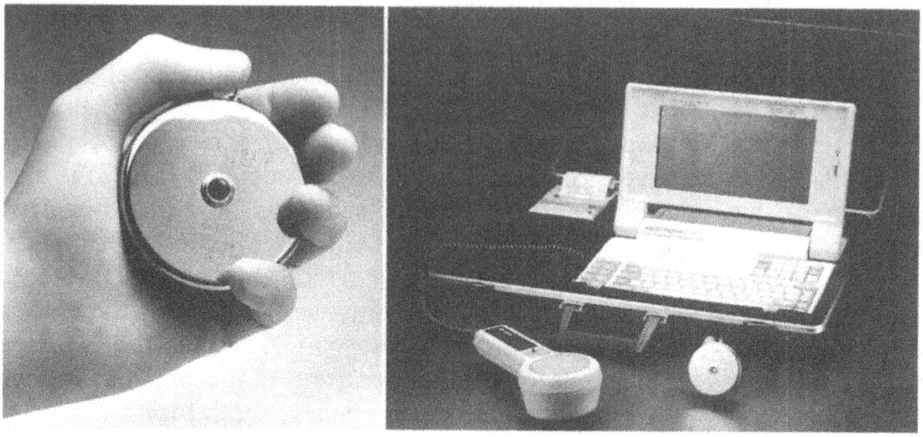

Fig. 4. The Synchromed[tm] infusion system from Medtronic: implantable drug pump and desk-top programmer

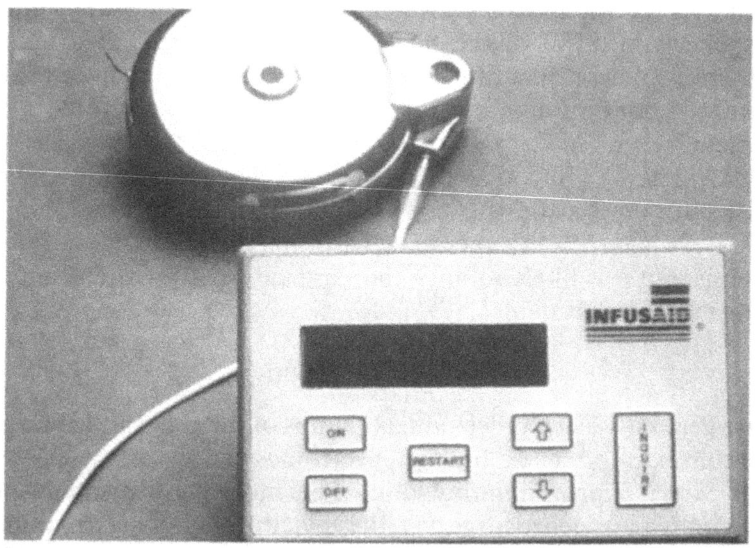

Fig. 5. The Infusaid programmable pump and portable programmer

the flow rate at the tip of the catheter is ± 15% over a temperature range of 35 °C to 42 °C. The infusion can be programmed in various modes: continuous hourly infusion, repeated bolus infusion with a specified delay, multistep dose over a programmed interval, or single bolus infusion. Although the rate of infusion can be programmed, the only way of stopping the infusion is via the remote-control module. This means that the patient either has to go back to the hospital where the device was implanted or go to a hospital equipped with the relevant programming unit. This is a major disadvantage, and it is a pity that there is no provision for the patient himself to switch the pump on or off. We have instructed all our patients equipped with this system, especially those that live far from the hospital or that travel widely, on how to drain and rinse out the reservoir with sterile saline in an emergency. Even after drainage, the pump will continue to infuse drug contained in the dead space, and patients must be aware that drainage of the reservoir will not stop infusion immediately. In addition, even when the pump is programmed to stop, the motor idles and infusion will still continue, albeit at a low flow rate (0.00018 ml/h). In practice this does not present any risk to the patient.

Infusaid have recently developed their own implantable programmable pump, the model 1000 (Fig. 5). It is quite large (90.2 mm diameter, 22.5–26.7 mm deep, empty weight 272 g) with a useable capacity of 22 ml. It is also equipped with a side-port. It is derived from the model 400 as it is also powered by the expansion of an inert gas (Freon) through flexible metal bellows. However, the output flow rate is regulated by a system of battery-powered, electronically controlled valves. Flow rates can be adjusted between 0.001 and 0.5 ml/h as periodic flow, multiple flow rates or as a single bolus infusion. The programming unit is miniaturized and portable, which increases patient comfort and safety. Unfortunately, it is rather costly, and this must be taken into account in the overall context of health care expenditure.

2. Implantation Techniques

Subcutaneous implantation can usually be carried out under local or neuroleptic anaesthesia. However, implantation of a spinal catheter can be carried out by laminectomy, and in spastic patients, it is generally preferable to perform the operation under general anaesthesia. The surgical technique is straightforward and will not be discussed in detail here. It has been described in numerous publications[60, 63, 64, 65, 68, 70, 71]. Nevertheless, it should not be regarded as a minor operation. Strict asepsis must be maintained at all times, and the positioning and permeability of the catheter must be checked carefully. A convenient point of connection to the access port or pump must be made available, and there must be a perfect seal between the system and the infusion catheter. The numerous complications (displacement of the implant, kinking or stenosis of catheter, fistula or accumulation of CSF, disconnection or subcutaneous leakage of drug, sepsis, meningitis, ets.) which may arise, can be avoided by the use of high quality materials and a rigorous technique. It is thus particularly important to check every step of the procedure to avoid technical complications which are not intrinsic to either the method or its application.

2.1 Catheter Placement

The technique depends of the site: spinal, intraventricular or intraarterial. The catheter is passed under local anesthetics or neuroleptanalgesia and under radioscopic control to determine its exact location.

A 14 G or a 16 G Touhy needle permits to place the intra-spinal catheter into the subarachnoid space. We use a percutaneous lumbar lateromedian approach so that the puncture pathway is as oblique as possible in order to avoid catheter kinkage during interlaminar penetration of the vertebral canal. It is extremely important that the connection is leak-free to prevent CSF fistulas and subcutaneous drug leakage.

The intraventricular implantation is done via a classical ventricular puncture. The distal tip of the catheter is either placed in the frontal horn of the right lateral ventricle close to the foramen of Monro or in the third ventricle.

2.2 Implantation of a Drug Administration System

Regardless of whether you are using an access port or a pump make sure that the pocket is situated 2–3 cm beyond the incision, not directly on top of it, but yet close enough fo facilitate fixation and to control the catheter connection. The subcutaneous surface must be thick enough to prevent skin necrosis especially with large-size pumps; but on the other hand, the system must not be implanted too deeply in order to facilitate transcutaneous palpation (filling, tactile feed-back, ...). Each system has its own particularities:

The access port. The entire system (catheter-connector-reservoir) should be as straight as possible in order to avoid kinks and assure optimal permeability. Before fixing the access port in the subcutaneous pocket the permeability is tested. For reservoir puncture, a 25 G needle will preserve the self-sealing properties of the septum. During chronic drug administration, the permeability of the system is controlled by observing a CSF reflux, by taking CSF samples for bacteriological analysis and/or by opaque solution injection, if necessary. Drug injection must be done slowly; once the needle is removed, and, if possible the septum is pushed down so that the bolus is progressively ejected into the subarachnoid space. The reservoir can be rinsed with an additional 1–2 ml bolus of CSF which has been drawn prior to injection of the drug.

The mechanical multidose pumps (Secor I and II, Cordis). Its fairly large size requires implantation on the lower latero-thoracic level for intraspinal administration, while the subclavicular level is more suitable for intraventricular administration. Before connecting the reservoir, we must purge it of all air bubbles by filling it with a sterile saline solution. The pump must per-operatively calibrated to check the bolus volume (0.1 ml + 10%) and filled with the drug solution.

The programmable drug administration device (Synchromed, Medtronic). Prior to implantation, remove all water in the reservoir and fill it up with 20 cc of drug solution in a sterile manner. Using the programmer under sterile conditions, we can then proceed with the examination and programmation. We must feed in data concerning the patient, the metrology and the nature of the drug to be administered (baclofen, morphine, antimitotics, saline solution, etc). The limits of the "empty reservoir" alarm must then be set. In practive, according to the pumps specific flow rate, we must program the quantity of drug that can be consumed before the audible alarm rings. At this point, the pump is submerged in 37 °C water to check if all the bubbles have been completely evacuated. Considering the pumps large size, it is preferable to make the subcutaneous pocket in the flank of in the para-umbilical abdominal area. The pump is now ready to be programmed. The programmer includes a computer-type console television screen, keyboard and transmission head. Programming is simplified by the fact that the software guides the manipulator, eliminating any chance of error.

3. Current Clinical Applications

Over the last decade, the use of implantable drug delivery systems has seen considerable development for the treatment of intractable pain and severe spasticity. There are now sufficient clinical data to determine their place in the treatment of these conditions.

3.1 Intrathecal Spinal and/or Intra-cerebro-ventricular Morphine in Intractable Cancer Pain

This was the first application of DDS in the central nervous system. It is based on fundamental understanding in neurochemistry and considerable experimental evidence.

3.1.1 Neurobiological Basis

A series of recent reports concerning the direct action of morphine on both the spinal cord[19, 32] and brain[1, 49, 73, 75, 116, 119], along with the discovery[42, 52, 98, 111] and localization[2, 3] of specific opiate binding sites and endogenous ligands has spurred development of new therapies for chronic pain, such as intrathecal morphinotherapy. This is the direct administration of opiates, especially morphine, into the perispinal and intraventricular cerebro-spinal fluid. Animal studies have shown that administration of morphine directly to the cerebrospinal fluid produces an intense and durable analgesia which is localized, dose-dependent, stereospecific and naloxone-reversible[119, 120]. These studies paved the way for the clinical use of intrathecal morphine[44,

[46, 80, 88, 90, 117]. It is mainly indicated for intractable cancer pain in the lower half of the body. With spinal administration, the analgesic effect has a limited distribution, and there is less risk of central respiratory depression than when treatment is given for pain of diffuse or cervico-cephalic origin. The existence of intracerebral opiate receptors[3, 98, 113], especially around the walls of the third and fourth ventricles, and the analgesic action of intracerebral micro-injections of morphine[1, 30, 116], has encouraged various workers to try direct intraventricular administration of morphine in humans[10, 69, 72, 74, 76, 86, 101, 115]. The efficiency, specificity and risks of spinal and intraventricular administration of opiates have now been evaluated in a number of clinical studies[64, 68, 72, 86].

3.1.2 Selection Criteria

Indications for this route of administration of morphine are based on clinical criteria backed up by results of intrathecal tests. Inclusion criteria are the existence of pain:

a) of a chronic nature due to inoperable, invasive and generally terminal cancer,

b) resulting from excess nocioceptive stimulation,

c) resistant to standard medical treatment such as administration of progressive doses of analgesics according to WHO guidelines. These patients must be either inadequately relieved and/or have adverse reactions to prolonged administration of morphine or its derivatives via the systemic, subcutaneous or oral routes (using oral solutions such as Brompton cocktail or slow-release formulations such as MS-Contin®),

d) with a bilateral, median and/or diffuse distribution, that cannot be relieved by surgical section of nocioceptive pathways (especially cervical cordotomy),

e) that can be relieved significantly by intrathecal administration of morphine.

The exclusion criteria are:

a) pain from sensory deafferentation such as post-root lesions of the brachial plexus, pain which does not respond to morphine or derivatives whatever the route of administration,

b) patients who have not received adequate doses of morphine via the oral route,

c) temporary or permanent contra-indication to implantation such as infection, suppurating bed-sores, coagulation disorders, etc.,

d) lack of consent from patient or family,

e) absence of a suitable medical or family environment for out-patient treatment and follow-up.

Two sites of intrathecal administration are used: lumbar puncture to spinal CSF, and directly into the cerebral ventricles. They are complementary, and their indications will depend essentially on the origin of the pain (subdiaphragmatic or otherwise).

3.1.3 Intrathecal Administration of Opiates via the Lumbar Route

This route is preferred for treatment of intractable cancer pain involving the lower half of the body. We will describe our experience, and discuss it in relation to other reports in the literature.

Patients

Between September 1978 and March 1990, 128 patients (76 male, 56 female) were selected for chronic spinal administration. The mean age was 61 years with a range of 35 to 80 years. All had become tolerant to oral or parenteral opiate agonists (60 to 300 mg/24 h; mean, 100 mg oral morphine/24 h). The duration of intractable pain before intrathecal administration ranged from 2 to 60 months (mean, 8 months).

The distribution of the primary malignant tumours was as follows: 73 pelvic (rectum 26, kidney 13, bladder 8, uterus 13, sacrum 2, prostate 11), 26 abdominal (colon 9, stomach 5, pancreas 11, retro-peritoneal leimyosarcoma 1), 9 cervico-thoracic (larynx 1, breast 3, lung 5). In 76 cases, the pain was secondary to regional involvement of lumbosacral plexuses. In others, the problem was essentially due to bone metastases (30 cases), visceral metastases (10 cases), or mixed lesions with invasion and metastases (12 cases).

Implantation Technique

The details concerning the implantation technique under local or neuroleptic analgesia are described in section 2.

Morphine solution and administration technique: The preservative-free morphine administered was a hyperbaric solution (7% dextrose) at a concentration of 5 mg/ml. Reservoir puncture was carried out using a fine needle (25 G) in a sterile technique. To check that the system is functioning correctly, 2 ml of cerebrospinal fluid (CSF) are withdrawn and retained for subsequent flushing of the reservoir after the morphine injection. The bolus of morphine is administered slowly into the reservoir. A 0.22 mm Millipore filter can be inserted between the syringe and the needle to ensure that the solution is free of bacteria. Serial CSF samples are then drawn for chemical and bacteriological analyses.

After administration, the patients were maintained in a 40–60 ° head-up position for 4 to 6 hours under routine cardiorespiratory monitoring (apnea monitoring). Nursing staff must be prepared to reverse any occurrence of respiratory depression promptly with naloxone.

A low dose of morphine is given initially (2.5 mg). The doses are then progressively increased (5 mg, 7.5 mg, etc.) depending on the analgesia produced.

Results

Evaluation criteria: Analgesia was evaluated using a multifactorial clinical approach[63, 65, 69], based on the estimation of three pain-related criteria: 1) pain relief graded using a subjective linear scale; 2) impact on the patient's level of activity; (3) consumption of other analgesic drugs. Taken together, these three criteria provide a semi-quantitative evaluation of the analgesia obtained in any given patient. Side effects due to direct chronic spinal administration, such as central depression and tolerance, were monitored and noted as well as complications resulting from the implantation. One of us (B. S-C) was responsible for instructing the patient, the family members, and/or the nurses in charge of the out-patient treatment. She was also responsible for keeping in contact with them and their general physician.

Clinical response: The mean follow-up period for this series of 127 patients was 98 days (range 8–913). The mean initial daily dose of morphine was 2.5 mg (range 1.0–7.5 mg). All the patients reported significant analgesia within 5–20 min (mean latency 10 minutes), and pain relief lasted from 6 to 96 hours (mean, 32 h). During the course of treatment, the daily doses of morphine were increased moderately with a mean terminal daily dose of 5.5 mg (range 1.0 to 60 mg).

The final results (concerning the 127 now deceased patients) are: 102 cases of good and excellent results (80%), 21 moderate results (16.5%) and 4 failures (3%) with a mean follow-up of 3 months. We only observed two cases of significant tolerance. For one patient, the daily dose had to be increased from 2.5 mg to 60 mg to produce sufficient analgesia for a follow-up period of 159 days. For the other patient, the dose was increased from 2.5 mg to 50 mg over a 197 day follow-up period.

Fourteen other patients required a moderate increase in daily morphine [10 mg (10 cases), 15 mg (3 cases) and 20 mg (1 case)]. In the majority of cases (86%), analgesia was stable during the total follow-up period.

Side Effects of Morphine

Table 1 summarizes the side effects during the total follow-up (initial trial, titration period, and chronic administration).

The most common side effects were nausea and vomiting (45/128). The nausea generally subsided. In addition, 8 males presented urinary retention,

Table 1. *Morphine Side Effects After Lumbar Spinal Administration* (n = 128)

Nausea, vomiting	45
Constipation	1
Urinary retention	8
Dizziness	1
Drowsiness	12
Respiratory depression	5

which was transient in 7 cases. In one patient with a "bladder tumour", we replaced the morphine with an agonist, buprenorphin.

None of the patients, and in particular those in whom the follow-up was longest, developed any neurotoxic disorders secondary to the chronic intrathecal injection of morphine.

We saw 5 cases of central depression with drowsiness, myosis and respiratory disturbances. Three occurred during the initial test: in one case after administration of 5 mg of isobaric morphine at Th12, in another case after administration in the epidural space at Th6, and in the last case, after administration of 2 mg of isobaric morphine at Th5. These three spontaneously reversible complications did not require intubation or naloxone.

The fourth complication developed slowly in an out-patient implanted with a pump programmed to a continuous flow of 3.1 mg/day. The somnolence and respiratory depression were immediately reversed by naloxone. The pump was reprogrammed to a 2.5 mg/day bolus delay regimen without further incident. The fifth case occurred during the chronic administration period. The patient received 50 mg instead of 5 mg. This required intubation, and injection of naloxone.

In this series of 128 patients, we only had two local infections of the implant which had to be removed in one case. Purulent meningitis occurred in 8 cases, 4 during the initial trial, and 4 during chronic administration. In one case, the implant had to be removed. The others recovered after intrathecal administration of antibiotics via the implanted reservoir.

Discussion

In 128 patients suffering from chronic cancer pain intractable to oral or parenteral opiates (mean, 115 mg oral morphine per day), we obtained significant analgesia with low doses of morphine (1.0 mg to 7.5 mg) via the intrathecal route. There was a latency period of between 5 and 20 minutes, and pain relief lasted between 24 and 72 hours. Use of an hyperbaric solution of morphine (7% dextrose) increased the mean duration of analgesia[17]. These values are in good agreement with those of other authors[18, 25, 37, 78, 127]. The distribution of analgesia was metameric with a maximal caudal effect.

Among the 128 patients treated with spinal morphine, only 8 cases had thoracic or cervical cancer, but the location of the pain was always subdiaphragmatic, stemming from lumbosacral and iliac bone metastasis. In one case with cancer of the larynx and cervico-thoracic metastases, pain was only partially relieved after intrathecal morphine administration.

During the follow-up period (mean, 98 days) a steady increase in the daily doses (mean, 2.5 mg at the start and 5.5 mg at the end of the treatment) was needed to maintain the analgesic effects. These doses are comparable to those reported by other workers.

Transient siede effects such as nausea and vomiting, skin reactions and itching occurred frequently in the initial period of the treatment[33, 72, 86]. Transient urinary retention appears to be specific to spinal administration[68, 72, 90], while behavior disorders or mood swings are not observed.

The risk of central respiratory depression is low, as patients had already received significant amounts of oral or parenteral morphine. We noted 5 cases of respiratory depression. In three cases, central depressant complications occurred after intrathecal administration of an isobaric morphine solution as also reported by others[40]. In agreement with other authors[105, 125], we found that depressant effects may be reduced by administration of morphine in an hyperbaric solution with the patient in a 40–60 ° head-up position. In the other two cases, respiratory depression was due to overdosage. The choice between spinal intrathecal and intraventricular morphinotherapy will be discussed in section 3.1.4.

The future of this conservative and non-invasive method also relies on the development of new opioids activating different opiate receptors. During percutaneous intrathecal spinal screening, we tried the administration of pentazocine (5 mg) in 12 cases, and 1.13 or 1.10 amine dynorphin (100–200 g) in 5 cases. The results were disappointing. Recently, we have also tried buprenorphin in 11 patients during the initial period of intrathecal administration. The results were encouraging, and 5 terminally ill patients have been treated with this drug until their death.

However, use of this route of administration is in decline due to the introduction of new oral drugs such as Temgesic® (buprenorphin) or Moscontin® (slow-release morphine sulfate).

3.1.4 Intra-(cerebral)-ventricular Morphinotherapy

This is indicated essentially for pain with a supradiaphragmatic distribution such as that arising in cervicothoracic cancer, or the diffuse pain from metastases. This route of administration (ICV) can also be considered after failure of lumbar intrathecal administration for pain in the lower half of the back. We report our own results before discussion of the work of others.

Patients

From 1984 to April 1990, we selected 74 patients for chronic ICMV via an implanted access port. The age of the patients ranged from 40 to 80 years (mean, 62), and the duration of intractable pain before ICVM therapy ranged from 2–36 months (mean, 10 months). All were tolerant, oral or parenteral opiate agonists. The distribution of the primary malignant tumours and the distribution of the chronic pain were: 7 cases with diffuse bone or visceral metastases (2 kidney, 1 melanoma, 1 prostatic, 1 breast, 1 bladder and 1 vaginal); 22 cervico-cephalic cancers; 37 lung cancers with thoracic and upper limb pain; 8 abdominal or pelvic cancers. All eight patients with abdominal or pelvic cancer had sub-diaphragmatic pain, but there was a contra-indication or failure after spinal intrathecal administration of opioids via a lumbar access port.

Administration Technique and Morphine Titration

Using a sterile technique, the access port is percutaneously punctured using a 25 gauge needle connected to a 2.5 ml syringe. To check that the system is functioning correctly, 2 ml of cerebrospinal fluid (CSF) are withdrawn. This CSF sample is retained for flushing the access port after the injection of morphine. In case of doubt, the permeability of the device can be checked by injection of a contrast medium.

The preservative-free morphine sulfate solution (concentrations, 1 ml = 10 mg or 1 ml = 1 mg) is slowly adminstered from a 1 ml syringe. A 0.22 m Millipore filter can be inserted between the syringe and the needle to ensure that the solution is free of bacteria. Serial CSF samples are then drawn for chemical and bacteriological analyses.

In order to limit the risk of side effects and to gauge the efficiency, 0.125 mg of morphine is given as the first dose. Later, and according to the analgesia produced, the doses are progressively increased (0.25, 0.5, 1.0 mg, etc). The patients are kept under close neurological observation and cardio-respiratory monitoring (apnea monitoring) throughout this titration period. Nursing staff must be prepared to reverse any occurrence of respiratory depression promptly with naloxone.

Results

Evaluation criteria: Analgesia was evaluated using a multifactorial clinical approach[1, 20, 21], based on the estimation of three pain-related criteria: 1) pain relief graded using a subjective linear scale; 2) impact on the patient's level of activity; 3) consumption of other analgesic drugs. Taken together, these three criteria provide a "quantitative" evaluation in any given patient. Side effects due to direct chronic ICVM, such as central depression and tolerance, were monitored and noted as well as complications resulting from the implantation. One of us (B. S-C) was responsible for instructing the patient, the family members, and/or the nurses in charge of the out-patient treatment. She was also responsible for keeping in contact with them and their general physician.

Clinical response: The mean follow-up period for this series of 74 patients was 75 days (range 12–230 days). The mean initial daily dose of morphine was 0.30 mg (range, 0.1–1 mg). All the patients reported significant analgesia within 5–60 min (mean latency, 20 min), and pain relief lasting from 12 to 70 hours (mean, 28 h). During the course of treatment, the daily dose of morphine was increased moderately. The mean terminal daily dose was 1.7 mg (range, 0.1–20 mg). However, the relative increase was quite low, since the ratio between the initial and terminal doses ranged from 1.26 to 3.41. The final results (concerning 74 now deceased patients) are: 62 cases of good and excellent analgesia (84%), 10 moderate analgesia (14%) and 2 failures (2%) with a mean follow-up period of 2.5 months. We only observed two cases of tolerance. One patient had been totally pain-free with 1 mg of morphine 32 days before the trial, but progressive increases in daily dose up to 20 mg did not induce analgesia. For another patient, the daily dose had to be raised from 0.5 mg to 15 mg to produce sufficient analgesia. Eleven other patients only required a moderate increase in daily morphine, never exceeding a four-fold increase of the initial therapeutic doses. In the majority of cases (61 cases), the analgesia was stable during the total follow-up period.

Side effects of morphine: Table 2 summarizes the side effects observed during the total follow-up period (initial trial, titration period and chronic administration).

Table 2. *Morphine Side Effects After Intra-cerebro-ventricular Administration* (n = 74)

	Titration period	Chronic administration	T
Withdrawal syndrome	0	0	0
Constipation	3		3
Urinary retention	1		1
Dizziness	5		5
Drowsiness	8	1	9
Myosis	3		3
Respiratory depression	2		2
Disorientation, euphoria	6		6
Hallucination, agitation	1		1

Minor morphine side effects (nausea, vomiting, constipation, urinary retention, itching, dizziness, headache, disorientation, euphoria or drowsiness) were initially observed but were short-lived. Some patients presented multiple side effects. We observed three major central side effects during the trial and titration period. In two cases, after administration of 1 and 1.5 mg of morphine, resepectively, the patients developed drowsiness, myosis and respiratory depression. A third patient presented visual hallucinations and behavioral disorders after an injection of 1 mg. These three central complications were immediately reversed by systemic naloxone with only a slight decrease in analgesia.

In this series of 75 patients, we only observed 3 complications due to local infection of the implant. In one case, the implant had to be removed, while the other two cases with transient purulent meningitis recovered after direct intraventricular administration of antibodies via the implanted reservoir. No patient presented CSF fistula.

Discussion

The time-course of ICVM analgesia was rather variable with a latency period of between 5 min and 30 min (mean, 15 min), to give a maximum intensity between 15 and 60 min after administration (mean, 25 min). The analgesia lasted for 12 to 72 hours (mean, 26 h). These values are in agreement with those reported by other authors[9, 74, 76, 86, 115]. The analgesia spreads rapidly throughout the body, particularly clear-cut in the patients with diffuse pain from widespread bone metastases. This effect has been reported by all authors, and it confirms the animal data on analgesia induced by intra-cerebral microinjections[1, 31, 73] or ICV administration[12, 13].

During the follow-up period, repeated ICV administration required a steady increase in the daily doses of morphine (on average 0.30 mg at the start and 1.7 mg at the end of treatment) to maintain the analgesic effects. The average daily doses of morphine administered, as well as the range of doses used at the start and end of treatment, were comparable to those reported in the literature (see Table 3) for similar follow-up periods. Only Obbens *et al.*[87] report the use of much higher doses, between 3 and 60 mg/24 h for an average follow-up period of 92 days. The doses required depended directly on the doses of systemic morphine used previously. They also report a more frequent development of tolerance. These results conflict with ours and those involving larger series[10, 74, 77, 115] (Table 4). The risk of central respiratory depression with ICVM is low[76, 102, 103, 115]. We only observed it twice during the initial titration period over a cumulative total of 5000 patient-days. Drowsiness was also rare (9 cases, 8 of which occurred in the initial period), in spite of the high doses sometimes used by the end of treatment. Behavioral disturbances such as hallucination and nervousness, and mood swings were noted more often using this site of administration than after spinal administration[63, 69, 72, 86, 115]. Apart from initial and transient nausea or vomiting, digestive disturbances, constipation in particular, were short-lived, and ICVM did not have to be interrupted in any of the patients. We did not observe any cases of urinary retention which appears to be a directly spinal effect[45, 64, 68, 72, 80, 90, 117, 121, 124]. The lasting effectiveness and the low incidence of side effects are in general agreement with the literature data reported between 1982 and 1987[10, 12, 74, 76, 77, 86, 101, 102]. This is summarized in Tables 3 and 4.

In chronological order from 1982 to 1987, analysis of reports concerning ICVM shows that overall clinical experience, including our own, is still limited. Less than 300 cases have been published so far. Our disappointing experience with PVG stimulation[61] in eight patients suffering from chronic pain of neoplastic origin led us replace this technique with ICVM. In fact, in six cases with a significant follow-up period (3–12 months), there was a rapid development of tolerance (37 weeks) to deep brain stimulation which was not reversed of satisfactorily by simultaneous parenteral administration of serotoninergic drugs (L-tryptophan, 5-HTP or amitriptyline).Along with most authors[63, 68, 69], we believe that the choice between spinal intrathecal and intraventricular morphinotherapy depends essentially on the distribution of the pain. Table 3 shows that, excepting Obbens *et al.*[87], all authors restrict ICVM to the treatment of pain in the upper half of the body. Pain of this type generally stems from diffuse, cervicocephalic and thoracic cancers, or abdomino-pelvic cancers with metastases. The latter may not respond to spinal intrathecal morphinotherapy. How-

Table 3. *ICVM – Literature Data in Chronological Order*
A) Topography of Pain of Cancerous Origin

	n	Diffuse metastases	Cervico-facial	Thoracic	Abdomino-pelvian
Leavens *et al.*	4	—	—	—	4
Lobato *et al.*	44	12	19	4	9
Roquefeuil *et al.*	8	3	1	3	1
Nurchi	5	3	2	—	—
Thiebaud *et al.*	32	6	16	2	8
Lenzi *et al.*	38	5	29	4	—
Blond *et al.*	79	19	58	2	—
Obbens *et al.*	20	—	—	—	20
Lazorthes and Verdié	74	7	22	37	8
Total	304	55	147	52	50

Table 4. *ICVM – Literature Data*
B) Daily Doses, Follow-up and Results

	n	Doses (mg) min – max	Follow-up (days)		Analgesia (B + E) (%)	Tolerance	Side-effects	
			range	ave.			respir.	vigil
Leavens *et al.*	4	0.5–7	2–90	85	75	1	—	–
Lobato *et al.*	44	0.25–16	6–150	55	97	—	3	3
Roquefeuil *et al.*	8	0.4 – 7	8–120	73	80	1	—	2
Nurchi	5	2–4	8–48		100	—	1	—
Thiebaud *et al.*	32	0.10–15	4–230	50	90	9	1	6
Lenzi *et al.*	38	0.5–2	4–292	65	95	—	1	5
Blond *et al.*	79	0.05–3	3–132	65	94	—	2	—
Obbens *et al.*	20	3–60	7–510	98	> 50	+ + +	—	3
Lazorthes and Verdie	74	0.10–20	12–230	75	84	2	2	2

ever, for chronic pain of cancerous origin in the lower half of the body, we prefer, for both ethical and clinical reasons, to start with intrathecal morphinotherapy.

Although the effectiveness of the analgesia from ICVM is undoubied, the neurophysiological mechanism is still unclear. If the effect is purely supraspinal, we do not know which descending control systems modulate the input of the nocioceptive messages to the spinal cord[69]. It is thought that ICV-administered morphine acts directly on central structures rich in opiate receptor sites, and that these structures influence the descending pathways originating in the brain stem which inhibit neurons of the dorsal horn[12].

We feel that the intense and diffuse analgesia reported with ICMV is independent of any direct action of morphine which might have diffused to the spine. This is supported by the following observations:

1) The time-course and the topography of ICVM analgesia is different from that observed after spinal morphinotherapy[67, 69].

2) HPLC assay of morphine in lumbar CSF after ICV administration showed that perispinal diffusion occurs after the development of analgesia, and that the amounts diffused were not sufficient to induce direct spinal analgesia[8]. Thus, in a patient with two intrathecal access sites (one in the lateral ventricle and the other lumbar), repeated ICV administration of 1.0 then 1.5 mg of morphine did not lead to significant concentrations of morphine in spinal CSF 1 h after ICV injection.

3) The kinetics of ICV-administered radiolabelled iodomorphine showed that: (a) the radioactivity migrated very slowly, (b) after 1 h (i.e. after the maximum latency of development of analgesia) only 5% of the injected dose had left the cerebral ventricles, and (c) the drug did not diffuse beyond the thoracic region[114].

3.1.5 Conclusion – Perspectives

The use of morphinotherapy by intra-ventricular (ICVM) administration for treatment of chronic intractable pain of cancerous origin is supported by recent fundamental data. This new method has aroused considerable clinical interest not only because it is effective, but also because it is relatively non-invasive, and the drug effect is reversible. It now forms part of the panoply of modern neurosurgical techniques involving activation of neurophysiological control mechanisms.

In patients who have become tolerant to large doses of parenterally administered morphine, ICVM produces fast and complete analgesia at low doses. Tolerance with ICVM is reduced since the mean terminal daily dose is 1.5 mg in the various published series. Although the site of administration is central, the side effects, especially central depression, are moderate. They are generally observed in the initial period and are rapidly reversible. There is, however,a potential risk with this technique, and patients must be carefully monitored. The intra-ventricular route of administration is complimentary to the lumbar intrathecal route, and the choice of route will depend mainly on the site of the pain. ICVM is particularly indicated for chronic neoplastic pain of cervico-cephalic, thoracic or diffuse origin arising from widespread bone metastases.

3.2 Intrathecal Baclofen for Control of Severe Spasticity

3.2.1 Neurochemical and Pharmacokinetic Basis

For the last 20 years, Baclofen (Lioresal®) has been the most widely used antispastic drug, especially in the treatment of motor and spastic syndromes, notably of spinal origin[27, 122]. Its effect on the increased muscle tone and spinal neuron hyper-excitability is attributed mainly to its ability to block the release of neurotransmitters at spinal synapses[128]. Baclofen is a specific agonist of gamma-aminobutyric acid B receptors which are abundant in the superficial layers of the spinal cord[15, 16, 100]. When given orally, Baclofen does not readily penetrate the blood-brain barrier[55, 56], and it is distributed equally to the brain and spinal cord, giving rise to side effects at therapeutic doses, of which the most troublesome is somnolence. To get round these obstacles, Penn[58, 91, 92] pioneered direct intrathecal administration of this drug for the treatment of severe spasticity. This was aimed at direct activation of GABA-B receptors by preferential perfusion in the spinal cord in an attempt to limit the central effects.

3.2.2 Patient Selection Criteria

Clinical pre-selection was based on the following criteria:

Cases of severe invalidating spasticity secondary to a stable spinal cord or cerebral lesion itself secondary to:

- lesion of traumatic origin (para, tetra or hemiplegia),
- a demyelinating spinal disease such as multiple sclerosis specially in its slowly progressive spinal form,
- or a motor disability of cerebral origin with spastic predominance.

Failure of medical treatment, and notably of oral Baclofen administration over a protracted period. Usually, it is the occurrence of unacceptable side effects (constant drowsiness and confusion) which limits an increase in oral dose. In the present study, all the patients were taking around 90 mg of Baclofen (60–100 mg) per 24 hours in association with other anti-spastic drugs such as diazepam and sodium dantrolene without any effect on their spastic and motor syndrome.

Absence of contra-indications for pharmacological reasons (vis-à-vis Baclofen), or psychological or local reasons such as bed-sores or skin lesions in the lumbo-abdomino-pelvic region which preclude the percutaneous implantation of a catheter or drug delivery system. It is essential that conditions (limb bed-sores, urinary infections, etc). which, though they may not interfere with the implantation site, can aggravate the spastic syndrome, be treated before any intrathecal pharmacological trial.

Consent from the patient clearly informed as to the constraints of the method (regular consultations, adaptation of dose, etc.) and therapeutic limitations.

Finally, the patient must be in an environment (family, general practitioner or institution) that is favorable to regular follow-up as an out-patient.

After clinical evaluation, the definitive selection is confirmed by a test lumbar intrathecal administration of Baclofen. This preliminary trial is an essential step before considering chronic out-patient treatment. It is carried out in the homes of patients who satisfy the clinical criteria for inclusion, and is designed to test individual tolerance, to judge the efficiency of intrathecal administration, and to fix the effective dose of Baclofen for an 8–12 hour action. This test period often needs to be prolonged for several days, and sometimes for a few weeks. We therefore replaced the initial use of an externalized lumbar sub-arachnoid catheter by systematic implantation of a lumbar intrathecal access site (Cordis Multipurpose Access Port, or Miniport) allowing prolonged testing. The risk of complications (CSF leakage, headache from intracranial hypotension, meningitis, etc.) or secondary displacement using percutaneous sub-arachnoid catheters clearly increases with duration of the trial. Experience has also shown that it is preferable to wait for a few days, and even up to complete healing of the implant incision, before starting intrathecal administration tests. Simply implanting the catheter and the port can aggravate spasticity for several days, and thus affect the results of the first pharmacological tests. Progressive dose tests must be run as soon as the clinical condition stabilized. Whatever the previous oral dose of Baclofen, the first intrathecal dose must be low in order to evaluate individual tolerance. We usually gave a first bolus dose of 25 μg, and then steadily increased the dose, generally by 25 μg per day until a dose was reached which produced an effect for 8–12 hours. The test administration can be carried out either by repeated bolus doses, or by perfusion with a portable external pump. Clinical evaluation of the results by muscular testing is gauged by systematic exploration of the H reflex. At the end of the trials, the lumbar intrathecal access port was left in position. This was used for subsequent sampling of the CSF not only for cytobacteriological examination but also for pharmacokinetic study (HPLC assay) to check the steady-state intrathecal levels of Baclofen[104].

Out of 43 patients receiving intrathecal Baclofen, 21 were selected for chronic administration. Most of these patients (17/21) suffered from spasticity of spinal origin: 8 presented multiple sclerosis of the spinal form which was fairly stable, 8 others had spinal trauma, there was one case of spinal ischaemia secondary to a diving accident, and another case was secondary to transverse myelitis. The 3 other patients selected for chronic Baclofen treatment presented spasticity of cerebral origin: one case of cerebral palsy, one case of traumatic cerebral lesion and one spastic syndrome arising from hemiplegia of cerebro-vascular origin. The age of the patients ranged from 14 to 70 years (mean, 35 years). There were 12 men and 8 women.

Three of the first patients selected had been treated without success by chronic cervical spinal cord stimulation. Thus 22 spastic and motor syndromes tested by short-term intrathecal administration were excluded for chronic administration. The exclusion factors were either ineffectiveness of intrathecal administration or over-effectiveness with loss of useful spasticity of the lower limbs enabling the patient to stand and walk to a certain extent, or a reduction in residual motor performance of the upper limbs. Finally, other patients were rejected because of foreseeable difficulties in follow-up, or lack of conset.

3.2.3 Implantation for Chronic Intrathecal Administration, Titration and Out-patient Follow-up

We employed various implantable drug-release systems in this series of patients. The lumbar intrathecal access port used for the test was also used for chronic administration in the first 6 patients. This required repeated daily injections with its inherent inaccuracy in dosage and appreciable risk of infection. We have now gone over to implantable programmable drug-release systems that allow accurate administration of the titrated individual dose of Baclofen. The last 15 patients have thus benefitted from implantation of a Synchromed system. The implantation technique is simple, and can be performed percutaneously under local anaesthetic, although in some patients, implantation was carried out under general anaesthetic either at their request or because of excessive muscular spasm in flexion. The simplicity of the surgical technique of implantation does not, however, mean that technical precautions can be ignored, especially concerning the positioning of the subarachnoid catheter. The intervertebral space is generally punctured at the lower lumbar level (L3/L4/L5) in order to introduce the catheter far enough into the subarachnoid spaces to avoid secondary displacement. The distal end of the catheter under fluoroscopic guidance is usually placed at the level of the lumbar enlargement, i.e. between Th10 and L1. The exit of the catheter from the superficial lumbar layers must be carefully fixed to the subcutaneous or fascial tissue to avoid displacement and stenosis. The proximal end of the catheter is tunnelled under the skin, and linked to the drug pump which is implanted in a subcutaneous site, usually in the abdominal wall, but occasionally in a lateral thoracic position.

For safety reasons, the initial dose administered immediately after implantation was twice the effective 8-hour dose determined during the intrathecal selection test. Baclofen, supplied by Ciba-Geigy Laboratories as a intrathecally-administrable solution was used at 3 concentrations, either 50 μg/ml (during the test period) either 500 or 2000 μg/ml (during the period of titration and chronic administration). During the first weeks, the dose was steadily increased in steps of 10–20% of the daily dose depending on the clinical response and the effect on the H reflex. We observed a considerable inter-individual difference in the initial efficient daily dose (15 to 250 μg/24 h); mean, 90 μg/24 h). After determination and stabilization of the initial efficient daily dose, adjustments must be made periodically as a function of clinical response and incidence of side effects. This step is particularly important, and it relies on efficient coordination of the care team. A pharmacist in our team is responsible for liaison between our laboratory, the patients and their family and medical environment. The patients come in for regular consultations either as scheduled or if the alarm beep warns them that the pump reservoir needs filling within the following week. The residual volume that sets off the alarm system is fixed according to the daily consumption of the individual patient. Daily consumption increased moderately during the first months of treatment before stabilizing to an average of 190 μg/24 h (range, 26 to 500 μg/24 h). The maximum useful volume of the reservoir is 18 ml with a Baclofen concentration of 500 μg/ml. More recently, a concentration of 2000 μg/ml has been employed, so the period between refills varied considerably between patients. At each consultation, adjustments of the therapeutic dose were sometimes required in the light of the clinical and functional findings. The patients were informed about possible side effects, and the risks of overdose. Owing to the absence of antagonists specific for Baclofen, it is essential that the patients are aware of the first signs, i.e. excessive salivation, dizziness, nausea and/or vomiting, excessive muscular hypotonia spreading to the upper limbs, progressive difficulty in concentration with somnolence. A large overdose of Baclofen leads to respiratory depression and coma. Apart from a mechanical failure in the drug delivery system producing a sudden increase in delivery, overdose phenomena develop slowly, usually over a period of several hours or even days. If the patient is relatively close to the hospital, there is generally enough time for a forewarned patient and an informed family to come and have the dosage adjusted, or if necessary, the pump stopped and the reservoir emptied.

The clinical response was based on objective assessment of both the spasticity and the functional improvement. Spasticity was evaluated by scoring muscular hypertonus on Ashworth's scale[94, 97], although tendon retraction may hamper accurate evaluation. The frequency of painful spasms was noted during the clinical examination. Tendon and plantar reflexes were also determined. Functional improvement was evaluated on a scale scoring the different motor performances. The scale was derived from that proposed by Davis[29] for evaluation of the motor performance of motor invalids with cortical involvement. This scoring system was used successfully in a similar situation[110], and so we employed it to evaluate functional improvement. This was split into 3 levels: marked improvement (> 3), moderate improvement (between 1 and 3) and no improvement (0).

The Ashworth Scale

1. No increase in tone
2. Slight increase in tone, giving a "catch" when affected part(s) moved in flexion or extension.
3. More marked increase in tone but affected part(s) easily flexed.
4. Considerable increase in tone, passive movement difficult.
5. Affected part(s) rigid in flexion or extension.

Neurophysiological exploration of the Hoffman reflex (ratio H max/M max) was also employed to back-up the clinical assessment of hypertonia. This was measured using various procedures. During the test period, the H-reflex was measured before and after a bolus intrathecal injection. After implantation and during dose titration, the H-reflex was monitored semi-continuously during a rapid or slow infusion of the efficient therapeutic dose. Results were related to the clinical response. The H-reflex was also measured at out-patient follow-up in order to adjust therapy to individual functional targets, and keep the M max/H max ratio to within normal limits ($\leqslant 50\%$).

3.2.4 Clinical Results

3.2.4.1 Administration of a Single Intrathecal Bolus of Baclofen

Single bolus administration was employed during the test period, and only exceptionally during chronic treatment. In the latter case, the patient requires successive bolus injections (bolus delay) which assumes that the patient has reached his basal clinical state between two consecutive boluses. This rarely occurs in practice. In fact after a single lumbar intrathecal bolus, the latency of a clinical effect is relatively long (around 1 hour), and it affects the lower limbs first. Subsequently there is rapid development (about 15 min) with a drop in muscular hypertonia, progressive disappearance of tone and a somewhat delayed decrease in tendon reflexes. Babinski's sign, or the plantar reflex in extension, is the last to disappear. The intensity, the metameric topographic extent as well as the duration of the clinical effect depend on the dose administered and on the individual patient. The efficiency of an individual dose is based on clinical criteria since in some cases, full hypotonus of the lower limbs should be avoided in order to maintain "useful spasticity" of the extensor muscles.

3.2.4.2 Results After Chronic Administration

Our results only concern the first 18 patients selected and implanted for chronic intrathecal administration over the period from May 1984 to December 1988. The mean follow-up was 28 months (range 4 to 56 months). In all the patients, muscular spasticity improved significantly. All the patients were selected at clinical stage 4 (5 patients) or 5 (13 patients) on Ashworth's scale. After treatment for various lengths of time, all patients presented a decrease in muscular hypertonia: 4 patients at stage 1, 12 patients at stage 2, and 2 patients at stage 3. The improvement in spasticity was observed during the titration period, and remained stable thereafter. Moreover, an improvement was seen in 14 out of 16 patients with painful muscle spasms.

Functional improvement varied considerably between patients, and depended on both the clinical stage and the etiology. Long-lasting functional improvement was observed in 3 patients including a 26 year-old bedridden Th8 paraplegic who recovered full autonomy within the space of three years. He was able to carry out basic tasks, get about in a wheelchair and even to stand and walk with a walking frame. This stable improvement was induced by a continuous slow intrathecal administration of Baclofen (26 µg/24 h). Functional improvement was moderate in 9 other patients, although in 3 of them it could be regarded as a marked improvement. Treatment had to be interrupted in case 5, a 56 year-old C6 tetraplegic, despite an excellent initial clinical response, due to local sepsis complicated by transient meningitis. The access port had to be removed after 26 months, and there was some delay before a Synchromed system was implanted. Case 11, a 27 year-old complete Th4 paraplegic, increased autonomy and improved use of his wheelchair, but did not retain any residual motor function. Case 14 with minor paraparesis secondary to spinal ischaemia from a dividing accident, with effort-induced distal spasticity of the posterior muscles of the leg, was cured of the spasticity, but the initial handicap was slight, his functional category was not altered.

The last 6 patients showed no functional improvement. They were all severely handicapped, bedridden and presented with tendon retraction.

Improvement in these cases was gauged essentially in terms of nursing requirements. Four of these patients had multiple sclerosis. The most common etiology in our patients selected was spasticity of spinal origin either due to trauma (7 patients) or the degenerative myelopathy of multiple sclerosis (6 patients). Comparing the results obtained in these two subgroups of patients, the most significant and stable improvements were observed in spasticity of post-traumatic origin, especially the cases of incomplete paraplegia. In these patients, there was both improvement in the spasticity and functional gain. The only patient without functional improvement was a 29 year-old full C5 tetraplegic (case 7), although he had a reduction in spasticity with suppression of painful spasms, and thus an improvement in nursing comfort.

In the 6 patients with spinal spasticity secondary to multiple sclerosis however, the results were less favorable. Spasticity was consistently reduced and in some cases completely suppressed, but there was little actual functional improvement (good in 1 case, moderate in 1 case and nil in 4 cases). This lack of improvement stemmed essentially from the gravity of the initial state and the absence of residual motor function. Moreover, although the selection criteria used were those of stable demyelinating disease, this is a progressive disease and the spinal deficit is commonly associated with supraspinal impairment such as a cerebellar syndrome which augments the handicap. In addition these patients were generally referred to us at a late stage when they had become bedridden with irremediable tendon retraction which effectively compromised functional improvement.

3.2.4.3 Complications

Side effects may be of technical, neurological or pharmacological origin, and they represent a very real risk for this type of therapy. A rigorous methodology must therefore be employed with careful follow-up.

The technical complications included 3 cases with displacement of the catheter from the sub-arachnoid space towards the epidural or extra-spinal space. This occurred in patients implanted with access ports (cases 1, 2, 3). The initial sign of a complication was lack of effectiveness of the intrathecal Baclofen, confirmed by administration of a radio-opaque substance via the access port. In all cases, the catheter was repositioned with resumption of response to a previously established effective dose. Two patients, who were initially treated with a mechanically activated Secor pump delivering isolated bolus doses, had to have the device removed as there was imprecision in dosage. These patients (cases 7 and 9) were subsequently implanted with programmable Synchromed pumps with a successful resumption of treatment. Lastly, one patient, the only motor invalid of cerebral origin in this series (case 8), received an overdose due to a pump failure which led to respiratory depression and temporary coma. The pump had to be stopped in emergency and removed. In this case, the pump was a first generation programmable device (DAS system from Medtronic) which was implanted in September 1984, and which had operated perfectly for over a year.

Infections and Neurological Complications

We observed 4 cases of local sepsis around the subcutaneously implanted drug delivery systems, and 3 cases of temporary meningitis. There were no neurological complications. Of the 4 patients with subcutaneous sepsis, 3 were implanted with access ports (cases 2, 5, 6), and so required repeated daily percutaneous injections. The fourth patient, a case of severe immunodepressive multiple sclerosis (case 9) had a Synchromed system. Six months previously, she had developed temporary meningitis during a preliminary treatment phase via an access port. Although the implantable pump had not been implanted in the same place (abdominal instead of lateral thoracic site), secondary infection could not be prevented. The patient was bedridden and suffered from recurrent urinary infections.

Purulent meningitis was observed in 3 patients. This was treated by both local (via the access port) and systemic (i.v.) antibiotics. In 2 of these patients (cases 9 and 14), the meningitis established during the initial trial with the access port was isolated and there was no subcutaneous sepsis. On recovery, intrathecal treatment was resumed either temporarily (case 9) or permanently (case 14) via an implantable Synchromed pump.The third patient (case 5) developed purulent meningitis along with subcutaneous sepsis and removal of the access port was required before recovery took place. In this patient, who had an excellent response to intrathecal therapy, implantation of a programmable pump is planned as soon as the cerebrospinal fluid is clear of infection.

In summary, although the occurrence of local sepsis always led to removal of the access port and temporary or permanent interruption of intrathecal administration, the isolated occurrence of purulent meningitis did not stop the treatment program (cases 9 and 14). All the cases of infection whether local or meningeal were observed in patients treated via access ports. The increased risk of infection arising from daily percutaneous injections in immunodepressed patients finally led us to abandon this method of administration in favor of the now systematic use of implantable programmable pumps..

Pharmacological Complications

These represent an intrinsic risk of this method and are seen as an over-efficiency, an overdose, or a losee of efficiency due to acquired tolerance. Detrimental transitory muscular hypotonia was one of the most frequent therapeutic reasons for non-selection during the initial trial period. Some patients were rejected for chronic treatment, as the over-efficiency of intrathecal Baclofen abolished useful spasticity in the lower limbs, or reduced motor performance in the upper limbs.

In the initial titration phase, we observed muscular hypotonia in 5 patients. Three of these patients were treated via an access port, but we could not be sure that all or part of the dose had actually been administered, even though the access port was flushed after each administration. In two other patients treated via a Synchromed system, the transitory hypotonia was rapidly counteracted during the titration period. This highlights the necessity for exact tailoring of dosage. We believe that the required accuracy can only be achieved using programmable implantable pumps.

A minor overdose leading to diffuse muscular hypotonia with temporary drowsiness was observed in 4 patients, 3 of whom were being treated via an access port. This arose during the titration period, and did not recur during the period of out-patient treatment after establishment of the efficient daily therapeutic dose.

Serious overdose causing progressive respiratory depression and transient coma occurred in two patients. In one of the patients (case 8), this was due to malfunction of the pump. The coma and respiratory depression were corrected by respiratory resuscitation with intubation, repeated lumbar puncture and i.v. hydration to accelerate renal elimination of Baclofen. The pump was stopped in emergency and removed. Treatment was not resumed in this patient In the other patient (case 1), with advanced multiple sclerosis, the overdose occurred after a bolus administration of 200 µg of Baclofen into the access port. The moderate respiratory depression and coma reversed spontaneously without the need for respiratory resuscitation in intensive care. Accidents of this sort can now be avoided by interruption of intrathecal administration and i.v. injection of physostigmine.

Acquired Tolerance

After the titration period, the dose of Baclofen was usually adjusted every 24 hours. The dose increment varied greatly from one patient to another, although efficient stable doses were obtained within three months. We have yet to observe a genuine case of pharmacological tolerance.

3.2.5 Discussion

Our results confirm the efficiency of this type of administration in patients suffering from an invalidating spastic syndrome that in intractable to long-term oral anti-spastic therapy. All our patients had previously been treated with high doses of Baclofen (60 to 100 mg/24 h) in association with sodium dantrolene which in many cases was associated with diazepam. This treatment had become inefficient with side effects such as somnolence, and confusion.

3.2.5.1 Inter-individual Differences in Dose

The pharmacological tolerance observed during oral administration was overcome by intrathecal administration since very low doses could be employed. Typically, the therapeutic effect was obtained, after the titration period, for an average dose of 90 μg of Baclofen. We did, however, observe considerable inter-individual variation in threshold of efficiency (15 to 250 μg).

During the initial trial period with bolus intrathecal administration the effects of the drug were only felt after a latenty period of from 45 to 60 minutes. This was presumably the time required for Baclofen to diffuse passively through CSF to the dorsal spinal root junction via the Virchow Robin cisternae, and finally bind to GABA-B receptors in the superficial layers (Rexed, 1 to 4) of the dorsal horn. This is a fairly long delay considering that the anatomical distance is only a few millimeters. It may be a result of the low liposolubility of Baclofen. After the latenty period, the effects set in rapidly with a peak response 15 minutes later. We observed a decrease in the muscular hypertonia with a progressive disappearance of the clonus and the monosynaptic tendon reflexes and finally loss of the Babinski's sign. Muscle tone and reflexes can be entirely abolished with larger doses. Baclofen distributes rapidly in CSF, but to a variable height with a predominantly caudal, metameric action, depending on the local concentration. The duration of the effect is variable albeit dose-dependent, and symptoms reappear in the reverse order and just as rapidly. The effect is perfectly reproduced after a new administration.

These observations were reported after the first trials of Penn[91, 92, 96] and have been confirmed by various authors[43, 66, 67, 71, 81, 82, 94, 97, 110]. In the present study (n = 18), the follow-up period (on average 28 months) and the long-term results are sufficient to demonstrate a stable clinical response without acquired tolerance. In all patients, we noted that the 24-hour doses had to be steadily increased during the first month of treatment, remaining stable thereafter. The average efficient dose rose from 90 to 190 μg for a range of individual values between 26 an 500 μg. These results are comparable to those of Penn[93, 94, 96, 97] who found that in a series of 20 patients, the initial average efficient dose increased from 150 to 340 μg (range, 62 to 749). Müller *et al.*[82], in a series of 25 patients with an average follow-up period of 2 years, reported an increase in the average daily dose from 234 to 294 μg. All authors noted a marked inter-individual variability of the efficient therapeutic dose. In our series, it was of the order of 1 to 20.

Penn[94] reported a 1 to 30 ratio whereas for Müller and Zierski[82] it was 1 to 80 (10 to 800 µg). This variability can be accounted for by differences in enzyme-mediated metabolism, local clearance by recirculation, and range and extent of the spinal lesions. This stresses once again the importance of accurate dosage which must be carefully adjusted in accordance with the therapeutic objectives which will also differ from one patient to another. They depend on the clinical stage of the condition, and whether the desired effect is total abolition of spasticity in patients who have lost all motor activity, or partial reduction of spasticity aimed at conservation of a certain degree of useful spasticity in patients with some functional motor activity. In order to optimize dosage, we were guided, not only by the clinical response, but also by the quantitative changes in Hoffmann's monosynaptic reflex (H reflex) and CSF Baclofen levels.

The ratio M max/H max determined at each consultation, is an index of efficiency which may also be taken into account in the light of therapeutic goals. For example, after a bolus intrathecal lumbar injection (50 to 75 µg of Baclofen) to six patients with longstanding spasticity and impaired voluntary motor control, Latash and his colleagues[59] demonstrated that the dramatic suppression of the spastic signs was accompanied by more selective voluntary muscle activation. Tonic coactivation of the antagonists and distant muscle groups during voluntary contraction was decreased, while the agonist level on electromyography (EMG) was not affected (3 cases) or only slightly reduced (3 cases). Furthermore, in one patient with sufficient residual motor control, there was a considerable increase in the speed of fast isotonic movements, accompanied by the emergence of the ability to generate phasic muscle bursts on EMG that were characteristic of normal motor pathways. This suggests that Baclofen exerts different effects upon reflex pathways and descending motor pathways, and demonstrates that elimination of spasticity may also improve voluntary motor function in some patients.

3.2.5.2 Influence of Etiology on Functional Improvement

Analysis of the results showed that the efficacy depended on both the etiology of the spasticity and the clinical stage of disability. From the clinical findings and the results of the trials using repeated bolus doses, we found, in agreement with other authors, a greater effect on spasticity of spinal origin whether post-traumatic or secondary to demyelinating disease. In fact we found that the effect on spasticity and painful muscular spasm was more or less identical in the two subpopulations, but functional improvement was greater in trauma cases with spinal lesions, and in patients with stabilized neurological lesions and deficits below the level of the lesion. In multiple sclerosis, the progressive character and the associated spinal lesion of a higher level tend to enhance the handicap and reduce the functional improvement. The severity of the clinical stage also accentuates this difference. Initially, this therapy was restricted to the advanced, highly disabling clinical forms, such as bedridden patients or those with restricted freedom of movement. In these clinical forms, the motor deficit is complete below the lesion irreversible tendon retraction is common, and the only functional benefit concerns nursing comfort and suppression of painful muscle spasms. This was the case for 7 of our patients, 2 of whom had post-traumatic cervical or cerebral lesions, and the other 5 had multiple sclerosis.

Subsequently, patients with less serious clinical features were selected. In these patients, independence of movement and motor performance are reduced owing to the intractable nature of the spastic syndrome, and therapy is aimed at improving both comfort and autonomy. This is reflected by greater independence in a wheelchair with sometimes a real functional improvement in the motor performance of the arms, or walking with the aid of a frame, when there is residual motor function of the lower limbs with "useful spasticity". This was the situation for 8 of our patients, 4 of whom were suffering from spinal post-traumatic lesions at the thoracic level. For these patients, the functional gain was secondary to both reduction in spasm and improved motor control. Latash *et al.*[59] has also reported an unmasking of motor control by intrathecal Baclofen, although the degree of improvement does not appear to be predictable before intrathecal drug administration.

Future indications for this mode of administration will probably extend to minor clinical forms in fully autonomous patients with disabling effort-induced spasticity sometimes accompanied by painful spasms, especially at night. The problem here is essentially that of accurate dose adjustment in order to normalize muscle tone with conservation of adequate motor function and extensor tone for standing or walking. Dosage can now be adjusted with some precision using implantable programmable pumps like the Synchromed. Complex infusion cycles can be programmed allowing administration of higher doses at night to counteract painful spasm without interfering with motor function during the day. This was the case for two of our patients. In one of them, the distal effort-induced hypertonus was suppressed with no concomitant disturbance of motor function.

However, the spastic syndrome is not static, and numerous intrinsic factors (infections, asthenia, etc.) or extrinsic factors (changes in the weather, temperature, atmospheric pressure, travelling, etc.) can aggravate the condition, requiring temporary adjustment of the intrathecal treatment regimen. Although the implantable programmable systems available at present (Synchromed for example) can be programmed at the treatment center, there is no provision for the patient to self-prescribe a predetermined extra dose in the event of fluctuation in the spasticity.

The risks of direct intrathecal perfusion of Baclofen have been stressed by all authors, although technical risks should not be confounded with pharmacological risks. The mechanical complications were reported mainly during the initial period of development of the technique. Steady technological progress over the years has already solved many of these problems, and those remaining are likely to be overcome in the near future. We feel that access ports should be abandoned for chronic treatment, but they are indispensable for the prolonged trials during the selection period. We have also found it useful to leave the port in place during chronic treatment for removal of CSF samples if necessary. Along with other authors[53, 82, 94], we found that continuous intrathecal administration gave better results than administration by repeated injection. Of the 11 patients implanted with the Synchromed system, only one showed a better clinical response to daily bolus administration at a fixed time (9.00 a.m.). In the other patients, a better balance of the spastic and motor syndrome was obtained with continuous infusion.

3.2.5.3 Pharmacological Complications and Risks

Pharmacological complications represent the potential risks involved with this method, and they can detract from its value. Oral Baclofen is evenly distributed in the brain and spinal cord but its anti-spastic action is essentially at the spinal level. Increasing the dose via the systemic route thus leads to central side effects such as drowsiness, and confusion. Local intrathecal administration leads to a preferential perfusion of the spinal cord, although since the subarachnoid spinal and cerebral CSF compartments are continuous, central side effects can also occur with this route of administration. Our results, as well as the experience of others highlight the marked inter-individual variability in effective therapeutic doses (between 26 and 500 μg in our series), and the importance of optimal individual titration. This variability is accounted for by different rates of passive diffusion in both CSF and at the posterior spinal root junction, and differences in catabolic activity. There are also likely to be considerable differences in degree and extent of the lesions between patients. The half-like of Baclofen in the CSF is between 4 and 5 hours[96, 100]. In the event of an overdose, 30 to 40 ml of CSF can be withdrawn by lumbar puncture, or via the access port, for a quicker reduction in adverse reactions. Although it is not a specific antagonist of Baclofen, intravenous physostigmine (1 to 2 mg over 5 min) can counter its central effects, especially the drowsiness and respiratory depression[83]. It is therefore an effective antidote and improves the safety of the technique. However, it should be noted that physostigmine has a short half-life in CSF, and it may be necessary to repeat a 1 mg i.v. injection every 30 to 60 minutes. A specific antagonist Baclofen has recently been reported to antagonzie both the peripheral and central effects of Baclofen[54]. Delta aminovaleric acid has also been shown to have an antagonist action in the central nervous system[107]. The future availability of specific Baclofen antagonists will undoubtedly improve the safety of the technique.

3.2.5.4 Alternatives to Intrathecal Baclofen

Whether administered intrathecally or systemically, Baclofen is the most effective anti-spastic drug to date. However, during the percutaneous trial period (in 5 patients) and the chronic administration period (in 3 patients), we compared it to both morphine and midazolan. Intrathecal morphine has been proposed for control of spasticity[34]. With a follow-up period of 1 to 7 months, Erickson reported a significant response in spasticity of post-traumatic origin. Morphine is a non-specific opiate agonist of μ receptors. Its action is dose-dependent, selective, and it affects nociception and polysynaptic reflexes. Willer reported that intrathecal administration did not lead to any objective modification in the motor function or gamma monosynaptic reflexes in voluntary paraplegics[126]. In our series, we noted an overall decrease of spasticity, but it was quite moderate compared to the effect of Baclofen. In 3 patients treated over a 2 to 3 months period, we observed a falling off in clinical response, progressive urinary retention and acquisition of tolerance. We therefore discontinued intrathecal morphine whose only advantage is the availability of a specific antagonist, naloxone.

Midazolan is a water-soluble benzodiazepine that can be administered intrathecally, and it has been employed in the treatment of spasticity[66]. The clinical effect is moderate and rather short-lived as the biological half-life is around 2 hours. High doses provide no additional therapeutic effect and lead to somnolence.

The place of intrathecal Baclofen in the treatment of spasticity still remains to be established, while controversy still surrounds the surgical treatment of this condition[53]. Chronic electrical stimulation of the spinal cord has been used in the treatment of spasticity of post-traumatic origin or that arising from demyelinating disease[21], while stimulation of the anterior cerebellum has been applied in spastic and motor syndromes of cerebral origin[22, 29, 62, 123]. Chronic neurostimulation of the spinal cord or cerebellum is a conservative method, only slightly invasive, is totally reversible and is founded on neurphysiological principles[108, 109]. However, its immediate effectiveness is moderate with little clinical or neurophysiological response[89]. There is also a lack of appreciable long-term functional improvement. The relatively low efficiency of electrical neurostimulation led us to abandon it in favor of intrathecal Baclofen administration in the treatment of severe spasticity of spinal origin[109].

Functional neurosurgery for spasticity commenced as early as 1908 with the introduction of posterior radicotomy by Foerster. Since then, numerous techniques for interrupting the spinal reflexes have been proposed, including longitudinal myelotomy, or stereotaxic operations such as cerebellar dentatectomy or thalamotomy[109]. Apart from a chemical or surgical partial peripheral neurotomy, which is a viable option when only a single muscle group is involved, only posterior root section continues to be employed. This is not the classical general root section involving all the posterior rootlets, but rahter a selective rootler section at the posterior spinal root junction[111]. The aim is selectively to destroy the small nocioceptive unmyelinated fibers, and converse the large myelinated fibers which carry non-nocioceptive somesthetic information. This technique is thought to be a value for spasticity of a limited distribution involving the territory of 2 or 3 roots at most. This is especially the case for those spastic syndromes of the arm arising in brachial diplegia secondary to cerebral palsy.

3.2.6 Conclusion

There is now enough evidence showing the superiority of lumbar intrathecal infusion of Baclofen to oral administration and even to destructive techniques for treating invalidating spasticity of spinal origin[71]. In theory at least, its remarkable efficiency obviated the need for double-blind trials. However, in a recent double-blind crossover study (Baclofen against saline), Penn *et al.*[97] provided additional evidence that intrathecal Baclofen markedly reduces severe spasticity. The advantages of the method are that it is conservative, non-invasive, reversible and selective in that it can suppress muscular hypertonus and inhibit mono and polysynaptic reflexes without affecting residual voluntary motor function. Bedridden or wheelchair patients with longstanding spastic paresis can also benefit from improved voluntary motor function. A difficulty is the marked inter-individual difference in response requiring accurate determination of individual effective doses. Continuous microperfusion gives better results than repeated bolus administration. The treatment of intractable spasticity by this new technique will rest on a firmer footing when we have a better understanding of Baclofen pharmacokinetics. The availability of specific antagonists and implantable programmable pumps with adequate sized reservoirs that are both reliable and inexpensive would also be highly desirable.

However, clinical trials with longer follow-up periods are still required to assess possible long-term tolerance. We also need to establish optimal efficient doses that suppress detrimental spasticity without interfering with residual voluntary motor function in ambulant patients.

4. Other Clinical Applications and Perspectives

4.1 Intracarotid and Direct Intratumoural Chemotherapy for Malignant Glioma

4.1.1 The Rationale

The overall effect of antimitotic agents depends on achieving adequate concentrations at the tumour site over a sufficient period of time. The brain and the cerebrospinal fluid are limited access sites, and drugs delivered systemically do not reach the central nervous system in high concentrations. The carotid artery is the principal afferent for the majority of the supratentorial gliomas. It would thus be a logical step to employ regional perfusion of anti-mitotic drugs[24, 35]. Injection of equal amounts of ^{14}C-labelled BCNU via the intravenous and intracarotid routes in monkeys showed that 3-fold higher concentrations were obtained in the ipsilateral brain with the intracarotid than with the intravenous route. In addition, the perfused cerebral hemisphere received 4 to 5-fold higher doses than the contralateral hemisphere.

The advantage of intravascular chemotherapy is that it localizes the cytotoxic agent, and avoids local increases in plasma peak concentrations. High local drug levels for prolonged periods, and diffuse distribution of the anti-mitotic throughout the tumour boundary have been achieved in the post-operative intra-cavity chemotherapy of malignant brain tumours via an external catheter[14, 39] or implantable pump[47, 79, 93].

4.1.2 Local or Regional Intracarotid Chemotherapy

The indications are essentially cerebral malignant glioma (III and IV grade astrocytoma) with a unilateral hemispheric situation and secondary diffuse metastases. Surgical extirpation and conventional radiotherapy are carried out prior to chemotherapy. Chemotherapy is either given systemically following radiotherapy, or if there is a recurrence. The results of intra-arterial chemotherapy using various chemical agents in these indications have been lesenbed by various authors[41, 42, 99]. Some of these preliminary studies are listed in Table 5. Most of the authors have employed the femoral approach for each session of chemotherapy (normally every 2–3 months). The aim is to increase selectivity (supra-ophthalmic), in order to reduce the risk of neurotoxic retinal effects. Prior to chemotherapy, the blood-brain barrier can be rendered permeable by intravenous or even intra-arterial infusion of hypertonic mannitol followed by a rapid infusion of BCNU or cisplatinum.

Implantable pumps have been employed only by a few workers in this indication. In [99]1982, Philips proposed a slow, continuous FudR perfusion

Table 5. *Regional Chemotherapy for Malignant Brain Tumours*

Authors	Patients		Technique		Site	Drug
	GL	M	Cath	P		
Greenberg *et al.* (1981) Greenberg (1984)	30		30		I-A	BCNU
Dakhil *et al.* (1981)	7			7	I-V	Metho-trexate
Philips *et al.* (1982)	6		6		I-A	BCNU, FUdR, Cisplatinum
Feun *et al.* (1984)	20	10	30		I-A	Cisplatinum
Stewart *et al.* (1984)	16	16	32		I-A	BCNU, Cisplatinum
Beck *et al.* (1984)		3		3	I-Th	Metho-trexate
Morantz (1984)	11			11	I-T	Bleomy-cin

GL = Gliomas grades III and IV; M = metastasis; Cath = femoral catheter; P = Pump; I-A = intra-arterial; IV = intraventricular; I-T = intratumoural; I-Th = intrathecal.

(4.8.–6.5 mg/day) using an Infusaid 400 model pump for a 14–70 day period. A side-port was used for repeated bolus injections of either BCNU or cisplatinum. Ocular toxicity is the major complication with this method[42], and it appears to be related to the alcohol concentration in the BCNU solution. Supra-ophthalmic catheterisation should thus reduce the risk of retinal toxicity. The second toxic risk is purely neurological and is independent of the route (intra or supra-ophthalmic) or method of infusion. Nevertheless, implantable, continuous-flow pumps allow simultaneous infusion of such "cell-cycle-specific" chemical agents as FudR or even radiosensitizers (BUdR). Another advantage of these slow continuous-flow pumps is their ability to maintain high tissue concentrations of drug. In the near future, connection of a slow-flow perfusion pump to an intra-arterial, supra-ophthalmic catheter should become feasible without compromising patient safety.

4.1.3 Direct Intra-tumoural Chemotherapy

Intra-ventricular chemotherapy has been reported[26], while direct implantation of a catheter at the tumour site has also been envisaged. Local administration of cisplatinum to rats has been reported by Kroin and

Penn[57], although it seems that tissue diffusion (maximum of 2 cm) limits such applications. Local chemotherapy is tempting as it would considerably reduce the neurotoxic and other risks inherent in the use of such powerful drugs. Local microinfusion may be the technique of the future. Bleomycin has been tested in cases of glioma[11, 79], and other drugs have been tried via multiple implanted catheters[14, 39, 93]. Recently, Harbaugh[47] reported a phase I study of intra-tumoural methotrexate infusion in recurrent glioblastoma. This author showed that post-operative intra-cavity methotrexate infusion through a single catheter as well tolerated if systemic folinic acid was given to prevent peripheral side effects. Radio-immuno assay demonstrated that drug diffusion and levels in the tumour (biopsy and autopsy samples) and surrounding brain tissue (biopsy samples) was much higher than those achieved by systemic administration. At the present time however data on efficacy are not available from this phase I study, and no significant tumour response has been observed so far. Conclusions will have to await the results of further studies with methotrexate and other chemotherapeutic agents.

4.2 Intraventricular Cholinergic Drug Infusion for Alzheimer's Disease

Progress in understanding the neurochemical deficits of various degenerative diseases of the CNS has led to the development of new applications for local infusion of drugs. Recent data indicate that there is a reduction in cholinergic cerebral acitivity in patients with Alzheimer's disease (A. D.). Cerebral biopsies of such patients were also found to have reduced amounts of choline acetyl transferase (ChAT), a specific marker of cholinergic neurones, as well as a decrease in acetylcholine synthesis[23, 28]. Based on the possibility of a decreased muscarinic receptor activity in A. D. patients, Harbaugh *et al.*[44] suggestd perfusing small doses of muscarine agonists directly into the ventricular cerebrospinal fluid.

After toxicity studies in dogs, 4 A. D. patients were subjected to a preliminary feasibility test followed by a cerebral biopsy. A constant flow pump (Infusaid) was connected to a catheter placed in the lateral ventricle in 3 patients and in the cisterna magna in the other. Bethanecol chloride was infused slowly until the optimal therapeutic dose for each patient was obtained (between 0.05 and 0.7 mg/day). During an 8 months follow-up period, he observed a number of spontaneous, reversible complications: initial nausea, and in one case, a transient Parkinsonian syndrome which regressed after reducing the dose (0.6 to 0.4 mg/day).Although the therapeutic response seemed encouraging, experience is still too limited for any general conclusions to be drawn. Subjective family reports noted improvement in cognitive function as well as in the patients' functional capacity. Patients returned to their initial state after infusion of a placebo. The efficiency of this treatment has yet to be confirmed over a longer follow-up period with quantitative evaluation of mental function using standardized scales.

Since this initial study[44,45], Harbaugh[46] and Penn[95] have reported results of a double-blind study and escalating dose trials. They only noted moderate improvements in behavior and neuropsychological test scores after infusion of bethanecol, and they did not recommend treating this condition by infusion of any of the currently available drugs with implantable pumps. The prospects of this new therapeutic approach hinge essentially on neuropharmacological developments. In Alzheimer's disease for example, the goal is to find an agent that selectively reestablishes cholinergic activity. The possibility of supplying nerve growth factors directly to the brain of A. D. patients by intraventricular infusion has also been envisaged[50].

4.3 Intrathecal Infusion of TRH in Amyotrophic Lateral Sclerosis

The intrathecal administration of thyrotroping releasing hormone (TRH) in degenerative neurological diseases such as amyotrophic lateral sclerosis was proposed by Munsat[84]. It appears to be less toxic with a longer lasting effect by the intrathecal route than after intravenous administration. There is little information of date on the efficacy and the safety of this treatment, although a blind study is in progress[85].

4.4 Perspectives

There are many potential applications of direct CNS infusion of specific agents to treat neurological diseases or disorders. Systemic side effects, peripheral drug destruction, poor blood-brain barrier penetration often hamper drug therapy of such conditions[48, 70]. A number of trials can be mentioned:

Ballantine[6] has suggested that the intraventricular administration of lithium has potential psychiatric applications. Animal kinetic studies showed that intraventricular drug delivery can reduce both the extracerebral toxicity and the caudal neurotoxicity of lithium.

The intrathecal or intraventricular perfusion of anti-convulsant, glial 5-aminobutyric acid (GABA) uptake inhibitors such as THPO was suggested for the treatment of obstinate epilepsy[8, 48].

Intra-operative topical application of Nimodipine and post-operative intracisternal infusion of calcium inhibitors after repair of ruptured arterial aneurysms has been reported by Auer[4, 5]. Cisternal administration of Nimodipine (200 μg) was performed in 20 patients for 3 to 10 days postoperatively.

The use of L Dopa methylester in animal models of Parkinson's disease has been described by Hood[51].

Lastly, Harbaugh[48] has suggested the possibility of combining neural tissue transplantation with CNS infusion of neurotrophic factors.

Conclusion

Chronic intrathecal administration of opioids and Baclofen is now a routine therapeutic option for the control of pain and spasticity. The future prospects of local neuropharmacology are promising. They depend largely on progress in our understanding of the action of endogenous and exogenous ligands and the neurophysiological substrates of degenerative diseases. However, the neurotoxicity of new agents must be determined in rigorous animal toxicity studies before clinical trials.

From a technological standpoint, further developments in implantable and programmable drug delivery systems should be directed at improving reliability and safety, reducing cost and adapting the systems to patient needs. Over the coming generations, pharmacological neurosurgery is sure to see considerable development, and it represents a most promising field of research.

References

1. Akaike A, Shibata T, Satoh M, Takagi H (1978) Analgesia induced by microinjection of morphine into an electrical stimulation of the nucleus reticularis paragigantocellularis of the rat medulla oblongata. Neuropharmacology 17: 775–778
2. Atweh SF, Kuhar MJ (1977) Autoradiographic localization of opiate receptors in rat brain. I. Spinal cord and lower medulla. Brain Res 124: 53–67
3. Atweh SF, Kuhar MJ (1977) Autoradiographic localization of opiate receptors in rat brain. II. The brain stem. Brain Res 129: 1–12
4. Auer LM, Ito Z, Zuzuki A, Otha H (1982) Prevention of symptomatic vasospasm by topically applied nimodipine. In: Auer LM *et al* (eds) Proc 1st Int Symp Aneurysm surgery in the acute stage. Acta Neurochir (Wien) 63: 297–302
5. Auer LM, Suzuki A, Yasui N, Ito Z (1984) Intraoperative topical nimodipine after aneurysm clipping. Neurochirurgia 27: 36–38
6. Ballantine P (1984) Intraventricular lithium infusion and potential applications in psychiatry. In: A professional briefing on "Totally implantable pumps". Isle of Palms, South Carolina, Sept 19–22
7. Beck DO (1984) Continuous infusion of methotrexate therapy of meningeal carcinomatosis. In: A professional briefing on "Totally implantable pumps". Isle of Palms, South Carolina, Sept 19–22
8. Blackshear P (1979) Implantable drug delivery systems. Scientific American 241: 66–73
9. Blond S (1989) Morphinothérapie intra-cérébro-ventriculaire. A propos de 79 cas. Neurochirurgie 35: 52–57

10. Blond S, Dubar M, Meynadier J, Combelles J, Pruvot M, Vitrac P (1985) Cerebral intraventricular administration of morphine in cancer patients with intractable pain. The Pain Clinic 1: 77–79
11. Bosch DA, Hindmarsch TH, Larsson ST, Backlund EO (1980) Intraneoplastic administration of bleomycin in intracerebral glioma: A pilot study. Acta Neurochir (Wien) [Suppl] 30: 444
12. Bouhassira D, Villanueva L, Le Bars D (1986) Effects of intraventricular (i.c.v.) morphine upon diffuse noxious inhibitory controls (DNIC) in the rat. Neurosci Lett 26: 5410
13. Bouhassira D, Villanueva L, Le Bars D (1988) Intra-cerebroventricular morphine restores the basic somesthetic activity of dorsal horn convergent neurones in the rat. Eur J Pharmacol 148: 273–277
14. Bouvier G, Penn RD, Kroin JS, Beigue R, Guerard MJ (1986) Direct delivery of medication into a brain tumour through multiple chronically implanted catheters. Neurosurgery 20: 286–291
15. Bowery NG, Hill DR, Hudson AL *et al* (1980) Baclofen decreases neurotransmitter release in the mammalian CNS by an action at a novel GABA receptor. Nature 283: 92–94
16. Bowery NG, (1982) Baclofen 10 years on. TIPS, 400–403
17. Caute B, Monsarrat B, Gouardères CH, Verdié JC, Lazorthes Y, Cros J, Bastide R (1988) CSF morphine levels and analgesia after lumbar intrathecal administration of isobaric and hyperbaric solutions in humans. Pain 32: 141–146
18. Chauvon M, Samii K, Schermann JM, Sandouk P, Bourbon R, Viars P (1981) Plasma concentration after I. M., extradural and intrathecal administration. Br J Anaesth 53: 911–913
19. Conseiller C, Menetrey D, Le Bars D, Besson JM (1972) Effet de la morphine sur les activités des interneurones de la couche V de Rexed de la corne dorsale chez le chat spinal. J Physiol 65: 220
20. Cook WA, Weinstein SP (1973) Chronic dorsal column stimulation in multiple sclerosis. NY State J Med 73: 2868–2872
21. Coombs DW, Saunders RL, Gaylor M, Pageau MG (1982) Epidural narcotic infusion reservoir implantation technique and efficacy. Anesthesiology 56: 469–473
22. Cooper IS (1973) Effect of chronic stimulation of anterior cerebellum on neurological diseases. Lancet 1: 206 (letter)
23. Coyle JT, Price DL, Delong MR (1983) Alzheimer's disease: a disorder of cortical cholinergic innervation. Science 219: 1184–1190
24. Crafts DC, Levin VA, Nielsen SA (1976) Intracarotid BCNU (NSC-409962): a toxicity study in six rhesus monkeys. Cancer Treat Rep 60: 541–545
25. Crawford ME, Anderson HB, Augustenburg G, Bay J, Beck O, Benveniste D, Larsen LB, Carl P, Djeines M, Eriksen J, Grell AM, Henriksen H, Johansen SH, Jorgensen HOK, Moller IW, Pedersen JEP, Raulo O (1983) Pain treatment on out patient basis utilizing extradural opiates. A danish multicenter study comprising 105 patients. Pain 16: 41–47

26. Dakhil S, Ensminger W, Kindt G, Niedorhuber J, Chandler W,Greenburg H, Wheeler R (1981) Implanted system for intraventricular drug infusion in central nervous system tumours. Cancer Treat Rep 65: 401–411
27. Davidoff RA, Sears ES (1974) The effects of Lioresal on synaptic in the isolated spinal cord. Neurology 24: 957–963
28. Davies P (1979) Neurotransmitter-related enzymes in senile dementia of the Alzheimer type. Brain Res 171: 319–327
29. Davis R, Gray EF (1980) Technical problems and advances in the cerebellar-stimulating systems used for reduction of spasticity and seizures. Appl Neurophysiol 43: 230–243
30. Devulder J, De Colvenaer L, De Somer R, Dumoulin K, Rolly G, Capiau P (1989) L'administration d'opiacées spinales: revue de vingt patients. Douleur et Analgésie 11: 131–137
31. Dickenson AH, Oliveras JL, Besson JM (1979) Role of the nucleus raphe magnus in opiate analgesia as studied by the microinjection technique in the rat. Brain Res 170: 95–111
32. Dickenson AH, Le Bars D (1983) Morphine microinjections into periaqueductal grey matter of the rat: effect on dorsal horn neuronal responses to C fibre activity and diffuse noxious activity controls. Life Sci 33: 549–554
33. Duggan AW, Hall JG, Headly PM (1977) Suppression of transmission of nociceptive impulses by morphine selective effects of morphine administered in the regions of the substantia gelatinosa. Br J Pharmacol 61: 65–76
34. Erickson DL, Blacklock JB, Michaelson M *et al* (1985) Control of spasticity by implantable continuous flow morphine pump. Neurosurgery 16: 215–217
35. Fenstermacher JD, Cowles AL (1977) Theoretic limitation of intracarotid infusions in brain tumour chemotherapy. Cancer Treat Rep 61: 519–526
36. Feun LG, Wallace S, Stewart DJ, Chuang WP, Yung WKA, Leavens ME, Burgess MA, Savaraj N, Benjamin RS, Young SE, Tang RA, Handel S, Mavligit G, Fields ES (1984) Intracarotid infusion of cisdiamminedichloroplatinum in the treatment of recurrent malignant brain tumours. Cancer 54: 794–799
37. Fiume D, Piccini M, Tamorri M (1985) Two years experience of iterative intrathecal morphine for cancer pain. In: Besson JM, Lazorthes Y (eds) Spinal opioids and the relief of pain. INSERM Editions, Paris
38. Foerster O (1913) On the indications and results of the excision of posterior spinal nerve root in men. Surg Gynecol Obstet 16: 463–474
39. Garfield J, Dayan AD (1973) Post-operative intracavitary chemotherapy of malignant gliomas: a preliminary study using methotrexate. J Neurosurg 39: 315–322
40. Glynn CJ, Mather LE, Consins MJ, Wilson PR, Graham JR (1979) Spinal narcotics and respiratory depression. The Lancet 1: 356–357
41. Greenberg HS, Ensminger WD, Seeger JF, Kindt GW, Chandler F, Doan K, Dakhil SR (1981) Intra-arterial BCNU chemotherapy for the treatment of malignant gliomas of the central nervous system: a preliminary report. Cancer Treat Rep 65: 803–810

42. Greenberg HS (1984) Intra-arterial chemotherapy for malignant tumours of the central nervous system. In: A professional briefing on "Totally implantable pumps", Isle of Palms, South Carolina, Sept 19–22
43. Hankey GJ, Stewart-Wynne EG, Perlman D (1986) Intrathecal baclofen for severe spasticity. Med J Aust 145: 465–466
44. Harbaugh RE, Roberts DW, Coombs DW, Saunders RL, ReederTM (1984) Preliminary report: intracranial cholinergic drug infusion in patients with Alzheimer's disease. Neurosurgery 15: 514–518
45. Harbaugh RE (1986) Intracranial drug administration in Alzheimer's disease. Psychopharmacol Bull 22: 106–109
46. Harbaugh RE (1987) Intracerebroventricular cholinergic drug administration in Alzheimer's disease: Preliminary results of a double blind study. J Neurotransm 24 [Suppl] 271–277
47. Harbaugh RE, Dempsey PK, Nierenberg DW, Maurer LH, Reeder TM (1988) Phase I study of intratumoural methotrexate infusion in malignant brain tumours. Presented at the New England Neurosurgical Society Meeting, Woodstock VT, March 4, 1988
48. Harbaugh RE, Saunders RL, Reeder RF (1988) Use of implantable pumps for central nervous system drug infusions to treat neurological disease. Neurosurgery 23: 693–698
49. Hayes RL, Price DD, Ruda M, Dubner R (1979) Suppression of nociceptive responses in the primate by electrical stimulation of the brain or morphine administration: behavioural and electrophysiological comparisons. Brain Res 167: 417–421
50. Hefti F, Werner WJ (1986) Nerve growth factor and Alzheimer's disease. Ann Neurol 20: 275–281
51. Hood TW, Domino DF, Greenberg HS (1987) Possible treatment of Parkinson's disease with intrathecal medication: MPTP model. Presented at the New York Academy of Sciences, New York, NY, June 13, 1987
52. Hughes J (1975) Isolation of an endogenous compound from brain with pharmacological properties similar to morphine. Brain Res 88: 295–308
53. Kasdon DL (1986) Controversies in the surgical management of spasticity. Clin Neurosurg 33: 523–529
54. Kerr DIB, Ong J, Prager RH *et al* (1987) Phaclofen: a peripheral and control baclofen antagonist. Brain Res 405: 150–154
55. Knuttsson E (1983) Analysis of gait and isokinetic movements for evaluation of antispastic drugs or physical therapies. In: Desmedt JE (eds) Motor control mechanisms in health and disease. Raven Press, New York, pp 1013–1034
56. Knuttsson E, Lindblom U, Martensson A (1987) Plasma and cerebrospinal fluid levels of baclofen (Lioresal) at optimal therapeutic responses in spastic paresis. J Neurol Sci 23: 473–484
57. Kroin JS., Penn RD (1982) Intracerebral chemotherapy: chronic microinfusion of cisplatin. Neurosurgery 10: 349–354
58. Kroin JS, Penn RD, Beissinger RL *et al* (1984) Reduced spinal reflexes following intrathecal baclofen in the rabbit. Exp Brain Res 54: 191–194

59. Latash ML, Penn RD, Corcos DM, Gottlieb GL (1990) Effects of intrathecal baclofen on voluntary motor control in spastic patients. J Neurosurg 72: 388–392
60. Lazorthes Y, Gouardères CH, Verdié JC, Monsarrat B, Bastide R, Campan L, Cros J (1980) Analgésie par injection intrathécale de morphine. Etude pharmacocinétique et application aux douleurs irréductibles. Neurochirurgie 26A: 159–164
61. Lazorthes Y, Siegfried J, Gouardères CH, Bastide R, Cros J, Verdié JC (1983) Periventricular grey matter stimulation versus chronic intrathecal morphine in cancer pain. In: Bonica JJ (ed) Advances in pain research and therapy, vol 5. Raven Press, New York, pp 467–475
62. Lazorthes Y (1984) Chronic cerebellar cortex stimulation for grades spastic cerebral palsy patients. In: Davis R, Bloedel JR (eds) Cerebellar stimulation for spasticity and seizures. CRC Press, New York, pp 217–220
63. Lazorthes Y, Verdié JC, Bastide R, Lavados A, Descouens D (1985) Spinal versus intraventricular chronic opiate administration with implantable drug delivery devices for cancer pain. Appl Neurophysiol 48: 234–241
64. Lazorthes Y, Verdié JC, Bastide R, Clergue ML, Lavados A, Caute B, Cros J (1985) Chronic spinal administration of opiate: application in the treatment of intractable cancer pain. In: Besson JM, Lazorthes Y (eds) Spinal opioids and the relief of pain: Basic mechanisms and clinical applications, Vol 127. INSERM Editions, Paris, pp 437–463
65. Lazorthes Y, Verdié JC, Bastide R, Caute B, Clemente G (1985) Les systèmes implantables pour administration épidurale et intrathécale d'opioides. In: Besson JM, Lazorthes Y (eds) Spinal opioids and the relief of pain. INSERM Editions, Paris
66. Lazorthes Y (1985) Neuropharmacological en application intrathécale. Neurochirurgie 31 [Suppl 1]: 95–101
67. Lazorthes Y (1988) Chronic intrathecal administration of baclofen in treatment of severe spasticity. In: Müller H, Zierski J, Penn RD (eds) Local spinal therapy of spasticity. Springer, Berlin Heidelberg New York Tokyo, pp 215–222
68. Lazorthes Y (1986) Morphinothérapie intrathécale chez l'homme. Rec Med Vet 162: 1409–1419
69. Lazorthes Y, Verdié JC, Caute B, Maranhao R, Tafani M (1988) Intracerebro-ventricular morphinotherapy for control of chronic cancer pain. In: Fields HL, Besson JM (eds) Progress in brain research. Elsevier Science Publisher 77: 395–405
70. Lazorthes Y, Verdié JC (1988) Implantable systems for local chronic administration of drugs. Applications in neuropharmacology. In: Pluchino F, Broggi G (eds) Advanced technology in neurosurgery. Springer, Berlin Heidelberg New York Tokyo, pp 214–235
71. Lazorthes Y, Sallerin-Caute B, Verdié JC, Bastide R, Carillo JP (1990) Chronic intrathecal baclofen administration for control of severe spasticity. J Neurosurg 72: 393–402

72. Leavens ME, Hills CS Jr, Cech DA, Weyland JB, Weston JS (1982) Intrathecal and intraventricular morphine for pain in cancer patients. Initial study. J Neurosurg 56: 241–245
73. Le Bars D, Dickenson AH, Besson JM (1980) Microinjections of morphine within nucleus raphe magnus and dorsal horn neurone activities related to nociception in the rat. Brain Res 189: 467–481
74. Lenzi A, Galli G, Gandolfini M, Marini G (1985) Intraventricular morphine in paraneoplasic painful syndrome of the cervico-facial region: experience in thirty eight cases. Neurosurgery 17: 6–11
75. Lewis VA, Gebhart GF (1977) Evaluation of the periaqueductal central gray (PAG) as a morphine-specific locus of action and examination of morphine-induced and stimulation-produced analgesia at coincident PAG loci. Brain Res 124: 283–303
76. Lobato RD, Madrid JL, Fatela LV, Rivas JJ, Reig E, Lamas E (1983) Intraventricular morphine for control of pain in terminal cancer patients. J Neurosurg 59: 627–633
77. Lobato RD, Madrid JL, Fatela LV, Gozalo A, Rivas JJ, Sarabia R (1985) Analgesia elicited by low-dose intraventricular morphine in terminal cancer patients. In: Fields H *et al* (ed) Advances in pain research and therapy, Vol 9. Raven Press, New York, pp 673–681
78. Meynadier J, Blond S, Combelles M (1984) Treatment of intractable pain in patients with advanced cancer. Pain [Suppl] 2: S 344
79. Morantz MA (1984) Intraneoplastic chemotherapy in the treatment of primary brain tumour. In: A professional briefing on "Totally implantable pumps", Isle of Palms, South Carolina, Sept 19–22, 1984
80. Müller H, Borner U, Stoyanov M, Hempelmann G (1982) Theoretical aspects and practical considerations concerning selective opiate analgesia. Spinal Opiate Analgesia 144: 9–17
81. Müller H, Zierski J, Dralle D *et al* (1987) The effect of baclofen on electrical muscle activity in spasticity. J Neurol 234: 348–352
82. Müller H, Zierski J, Dralle D *et al* (1988) Intrathecal baclofen in spasticity. In: Müller H, Zierski J, Penn RD (eds) Local spinal therapy of spasticity. Springer, Berlin Heidelberg New York Tokyo, pp 155–214
83. Müller-Schwefe G (1988) Physostigmine reversal of baclofen-induced sedation. In: Müller H, Zierski J, Penn RD (eds) Local spinal therapy of spasticity.Springer, Berlin Heidelberg New York Tokyo, pp 253–254
84. Munsat TL (1984) Intrathecal TRH in motor neuron diseases. In: A professional briefing in "Totally implantable pumps". Isle of Palms, South Carolina, Sept 19–22, 1984.
85. Munsat TL, Taft J, Kasdon J (1987) Long term intrathecal infusion of TRH in ALS. Presented at the New York Academy of Sciences, New York NY, June 13, 1987
86. Nurchi G (1984) Use of intraventricular an intrathecal morphine in intractable pain associated with cancer. Neurosurgery 15: 801–803
87. Obbens EAMT, Hill CS, Leavens ME,Ruthenbeck SS, Otis F (1987) Intraventricular morphine administration for control of chronic cancer pain. Pain 28: 61–68

88. Onofrio B, Yaksh TL, Arnold PG (1981) Continuous low-dose intrathecal morphine administration in the treatment of chronic pain of malignant origin. Mayo Clin Proc 56: 516–520
89. Penn RD (1982) Chronic cerebellar stimulation of cerebral palsy: a review. Neurosurgery 10: 116–121
90. Penn RD, Paice JA, Gottschalk W, Ivankovitch AD (1984) Cancer pain relief using chronic morphine infusion: early experience with a programmable implanted drug pump. J Neurosurg 61: 302–306
91. Penn RD, Kroin JS (1984) Intrathecal baclofen alleviates spinal cord spasticity. Lancet 1: 1078 (letter)
92. Penn RD, Kroin JS (1985) Continuous intrathecal baclofen for severe spasticity. Lancet 2: 125–127
93. Penn RD, Kroin JS, Harris JE, Chiu KM, Braun DP (1986) Chronic intratumoural chemotherapy of a rat tumour with cisplatin and fluorouracil. Appl Neurophysiol 46: 240–244
94. Penn RD, Kroin JS (1987) Long-term intrathecal baclofen infusion for treatment of spasticity. J Neurosurg 66: 181–185
95. Penn RD, Martin EM, Wilson RS, Fox JH, Savoy SM (1988) Intraventricular bethanechol infusion of Alzheimer's disease: results of double-blind and escalating dose trials. Neurology 38: 219–222
96. Penn RD (1988) Chronic intrathecal baclofen for severe rigidity and spasms. In: Müller H, Zierski J, Penn RD (eds) Local spinal therapy of spasticity. Springer, Berlin Heidelberg New York Tokyo, pp 151–154
97. Penn RD, Savoy SM, Cordos D *et al* (1989) Intrathecal baclofen for severe spasticity. N Engl J Med 320: 1517–1521
98. Pert CB, Snyder SM (1973) Opiate receptor: demonstration in nervous tissue. Science 179: 1011–1014
99. Philips TW, Chandler WF, Kindt GW, Ensminger WD, Greenberg HS, Seeger JF, Doan KM, Gyves JW (1982) New implantable continuous administration and bolus dose intracarotid drug delivery system for the treatment of malignant gliomas. Neurosurgery 11: 213–218
100. Price GW, Wilkin GP, Turnbull MJ *et al* (1984) Are baclofen-sensitive GABA-receptors present on primary afferent terminals of the spinal cord? Nature 307: 71–73
101. Roquefeuil B, Benezech J, Batier C, Blanchet P, Gros C, Mathieu-Daude JC (1983) Intérêt de l'analgésie morphinique par voie ventriculaire dans les algies rebelles néoplasiques. Neurochirurgie 29: 135–141
102. Roquefeuil B, Benezech J, Blanchet P, Batier C, Frerebeau Ph, Gros C (1984) Intraventricular administration for morphine in patients with neoplasic intractable pain. Surg Neurol 21: 155–158
103. Roquefeuil B, Benezech J, Batier C (1985) Intérêt de l'analgésie morphinique par voie ventriculaire dans les algies rebelles néoplasiques. In: Simon L, Roquefeuil B, Pelissier J (eds) Le douleur chronique. Masson, Paris, pp 212
104. Sallerin-Caute B, Monsarrat B, Lazorthes Y *et al* (1988) A sensitive method for determination of baclofen in human CSF by high performance liquid chromatography. J Liquid Chromatography 11: 1753–761

105. Samii K, Feret J, Harari A, Viars P (1981) Post-operative spinal analgesia with morphine. Br J Anaesth 53: 817–820
106. Saunders RL, Commbs DW (1983) Dartmouth-Hitchcock Medical Center experience with continuous intraspinal narcotic analgesia. In: Schmidek H, Sweet WE (eds) Operative neurosurgical techniques, Vol. 2. Grune and Stratton, New York, pp 1211–1212
107. Schwartz M, Klockgether T, Wullner U *et al* (1988) Delta-aminovaleric system. Exp Brain Res 70: 618–626
108. Sedan R, Lazorthes Y (eds) (1978) La neurostimulation électrique thérapeutique. Neurochirurgie 24 [Suppl 1]: 1–125
109. Siegfried J, Lazorthes Y (eds) (1985) La neurochirurgie fonctionnelle de l'infirmité motrice d'origine cérébrale. Neurochirurgie 31 [Suppl 1]: 1–118
110. Siegfried J, Rea GL (1987) Intrathecal application on baclofen in the treatment of spasticity. Acta Neurochir (Wien) [Suppl] 39: 121–23 (1987)
111. Simon EJ (1982) Opiate receptors and opioid peptides: an overview. Ann NY Acad Sci 327–339
112. Sindou M, Fischer G, Goutelle A *et al* (1974) La radicellotomie postérieure sélective dans le traitement des spasticités. Rev Neurol 130: 201–216
113. Stewart DJ, Grahovac Z, Benoit B, Addison D, Richard MT, Dennery J, Hugenholtz H, Russell N, Peterson E, Maroun JA, Vandenberg T, Hopkins HS (1984) Intracarotid chemotherapy with a combination of 1.3-bis(2-chloroethyl)-1-nitrosourea (BCNU), cis-diaminedichloroplatinum (cisplatin), and 4'-0-(4.6-0-2-thenylidene-beta-d-glucopyranosyl) epipodrophyllonoxin (VM-26) in the treatment of primary and metastatic brain tumours. Neurosurgery 15: 828–833
114. Tafani M, Danet B, Verdié JC, Lazorthes Y, Esquerré JP, Simon J (1989) Human brain and spinal cord scan after intra-cerebro-ventricular administration of iodine 123 morphine. Nucl Med Biol 16: 505–509
115. Thiebaut JB, Blond S, Farcot JM, Thurel C, Matge G, Schach G, Meynadier J, Bucheit F (1985) La morphine par voie intraventriculaire dans le traitement des douleurs néoplasiques. Med Hyg 43: 636–646
116. Tsou K, Jang CS (1964) Studies on the site of analgesic action of morphine by intracerebral microinjection. Sci Sin 13: 1099–1109
117. Tung AS, Tenicela R, Bart G, Winter P (1982) Intrathecal morphine in cancer patients tolerant to systemic opiates. Spinal Opiate Analgesia 144: 138–140
118. Yaksh TL, Rudy TA (1977) Studies on the direct spinal action of narcotics in the production of analgesia in the rat. J Pharmacol Exp Ther 202: 411–428
119. Yaksh TL, Rudy TA (1978) Narcotic analgetics: CNS sites and mechanisms of action as revealed by intracerebral injection techniques. Pain 4: 299–359
120. Yaksh TL (1978) Analgesic actions of intrathecal opiates in cat and primate. Brain Res 153: 205–210
121. Yaksh RL (1981) Spinal opiate analgesia: characteristic and principles of actions. Pain 11: 293–346
122. Young RR, Delwaide PJ (1981) Drug therapy: spasticity. N Engl J Med 304: 96–99

123. Waltz JM, Reynolds LO, Riklan M (1981) Multi-lead spinal cord stimulation for control of motor disorders. Appl Neurophysiol 44: 244–257
124. Wang JK (1977) Analgesic effect of intrathecally administered morphine. Reg Anaesth 4: 2–3
125. Wang JK, Nauss LE, Thomas JE (1979) Pain relief by intrathecally applied morphine in man. Anaesthesiology 50: 149–151
126. Willer JC, Bussel B (1980) Evidence for a direct spinal mechanism in morphine-induced inhibition of nociceptive reflexes in humans. Brain Res 187: 212–217
127. Zenz H, Piepenbrock S, Hilfrich J, Husch M (1982) Pain therapy with epidural morphine in patients with terminal cancer. Spinal Opiate Analgesia 144: 141–144
128. Zieglgänsberger W, Howe JR, Sutor B (1988) The neuropharmacology of baclofen: In: Müller H, Zierski J, Penn RD (eds) Local spinal therapy of spasticity. Springer, Berlin Heidelberg New York Tokyo, pp 37–49

Author Index

Subject Index

Druck: Adolf Holzhausens Nfg., Universitätsbuchdrucker

Advances and Technical Standards in Neurosurgery

Volume 1

1974. 96 figures. XI, 210 pages.
Cloth DM 113,—, öS 790,—
ISBN 3-211-81218-0

Contents:

Advances: N. Lundberg, Å. Kjällquist, G. Kullberg, U. Pontén, and G. Sundbärg: Non-operative Management of Intracranial Hypertension. — J. Philippon and D. Ancri: Chronic Adult Hydrocephalus. — H. Powiertowski: Surgery of Craniostenosis in Advanced Cases. A Method of Extensive Subperiosteal Resection of the Vault and Base of the Skull Followed by Bone Regeneration. — E. Zander and R. Campiche: Extra-Dural Hematoma.

Technical Standards: B. Pertuiset: Supratentorial Craniotomy. — B. Guidetti: Removal of Extramedullary Benign Spinal Cord Tumours.

Volume 2

1975. 150 partly coloured figures. XI, 217 pages.
Cloth DM 125,—, öS 870,—
ISBN 3-211-81293-8

Contents:

Advances: J. Gawler, J. W. D. Bull, G. du Boulay, and J. Marshall: Computerized Axial Tomography with the EMI-Scanner. — M. Samii: Modern Aspects of Peripheral and Cranial Nerve Surgery. — A. Rey, J. Cophignon, Cl. Thurel, and J. B. Thiebaut: Treatment of Traumatic Cavernous Fistulas.

Technical Standards: M. G. Yaşargil, J. L. Fox, and M. W. Ray: The Operative Approach to Aneurysms of the Anterior Communicating Artery. — Valentine Logue: Parasagittal Meningiomas. — J. Siegfried and M. Vosmansky: Technique of the Controlled Thermocoagulation of Trigeminal Ganglion and Spinal Roots.

Volume 3

1976. 77 figures. XI, 154 pages.
Cloth DM 102,—, öS 710,—
ISBN-3-211-81381-0

Contents:

Advances: G. Guiot and P. Derome: Surgical Problems of Pituitary Adenomas. — H. Troupp: The Management of Intracranial Arterial Aneurysms in the Acute Stage. — Y. Yonekawa and M. G. Yaşargil: Extra-Intracranial Arterial Anastomosis: Clinical and Technical Aspects. Results.

Technical Standards: W. Luyendijk: The Operative Approach to the Posterior Fossa. — J. Brihaye: Neurosurgical Approaches to Orbital Tumours. — R. Lorenz: Methods of Percutaneous Spino-Thalamic Tract Section.

Advances and Technical Standards in Neurosurgery

Volume 4

1977. 66 partly coloured figures. XI, 154 pages.
Cloth DM 102,—, öS 710,—
ISBN 3-211-81423-X

Contents:

Advances: N. A. Lassen and D. H. Ingvar: Clinical Relevance of Cerebral Blood Flow Measurements. — G. W. Taylor and J. S. P. Lumley: Extra-Cranial Surgery for Cerebrovascular Disease. — J. Rétif: Intrathecal Injection of a Neurolytic Solution for the Relief of Intractable Pain.

Technical Standards: L. Symon: Olfactory Groove and Suprasellar Meningiomas. — M. G. Yaşargil, R. D. Smith, and J. C. Gasser: Microsurgical Approach to Acoustic Neurinomas. — G. Debrun, P. Lacour, and J. P. Caron: Balloon Arterial Catheter Techniques in the Treatment of Arterial Intracranial Diseases.

Volume 5

1978. 78 figures. XII, 224 pages.
Cloth DM 136,—, öS 950,—
ISBN 3-211-81441-8

Contents:

Advances: A. M. Landolt: Progress in Pituitary Adenoma Biology. Results of Research and Clinical Applications. — J. Hildebrand and J. Brihaye: Chemotherapy of Brain Tumours. — S. Mingrino: Supratentorial Arteriovenous Malformations of the Brain.

Technical Standards: J. Hankinson: The Surgical Treatment of Syringomyelia. — F. Loew and W. Caspar: Surgical Approach to Lumbar Disc Herniations. — B. Pertuiset, D. Fohanno, and O. Lyon-Caen: Recurrent Instability of the Cervical Spine With Neurological Implications—Treatment by Anterior Spinal Fusion.

Volume 6

1979. 79 figures. XI, 191 pages.
Cloth DM 125, —, öS 870,—
ISBN 3-211-81518-X

Contents:

Advances: E.-O. Backlund: Stereotactic Radiosurgery in Intracranial Tumors and Vascular Malformations. — J. Klastersky, L. Kahan-Coppens, and J. Brihaye: Infection in Neurosurgery. — C. Gros: Spasticity-Clinical Classification and Surgical Treatment.

Technical Standards: P. J. Derome and G. Guiot in co-operation with B. Georges, M. Porta, A. Visot, and S. Balagura: Surgical Approaches to the Sphenoidal and Clival Areas. — R. Braakman: Cervical Spondylotic Myelopathy. — F. Isamat: Tumours of the Posterior Part of the Third Ventricle: Neurosurgical Criteria.

Volume 7

1980. 147 figures. XI, 247 pages.
Cloth DM 139,—, öS 970,—
ISBN 3-211-81592-9

Contents:

Advances: M. G. Yasargil, R. W. Mortara, and M. Curcic: Meningiomas of Basal Posterior Cranial Fossa.

Technical Standards: A. M. Landolt and P. Strebel: Technique of Transsphenoidal Operation for Pituitary Adenomas. — Surgical Treatment of Facial Nerve Paralysis; Longterm Results: H. Millesi: Extratemporal Surgery of the Facial Nerve — Palliative Surgery. S. Mingrino: Intracranial Surgical Repair of the Facial Nerve. U. Fisch: Management of Intratemporal Facial Palsy.

Advances and Technical Standards in Neurosurgery

Volume 8

1981. 135 partly coloured figures. XII, 328 pages.
Cloth DM 172,—, öS 1200,—
ISBN 3-211-81665-8

Contents:

Advances: E. de Divitiis, R. Spaziante, and L. Stella: Empty Sella and Benign Intrasellar Cysts. — B. Pertuiset, D. Ancri, and A. Lienhart: Profound Arterial Hypotension (MAP ≦ 50 mm Hg) Induced with Neuroleptanalgesia and Sodium Nitroprusside (Series of 531 Cases). Reference to Vascular Autoregulation Mechanism and Surgery of Vascular Malformations of the Brain. — F. Gullotta: Morphological and Biological Basis for the Classification of Brain Tumors. With a Comment on the WHO-Classification 1979.

Technical Standards: E. Pásztor: Surgical Treatment of Spondylotic Vertebral Artery Compression. — P. Harris, I. T. Jackson, and J. C. McGregor: Reconstructive Surgery of the Head. — A. N. Konovalov: Operative Management of Craniopharyngiomas.

Volume 9

1982. 88 figures. XI, 177 pages.
Cloth DM 113,—, öS 790,—
ISBN 3-211-81718-2

Contents:

Advances: K. Faulhauer: The Overdrained Hydrocephalus. Clinical Manifestations and Management. — A. P. Romodanov and V. I. Shcheglov: Intravascular Occlusion of Saccular Aneurysms of the Cerebral Arteries by Means of a Detachable Balloon Catheter. — H. Spiess: Advances in Computerized Tomography.

Technical Standards: L. Symon: Surgical Approaches to the Tentorial Hiatus. — F. Loew: Management of Chronic Subdural Haematomas and Hygromas. — B. Williams: Subdural Empyema.

Volume 10

1983. 70 figures (1 in color). XI, 231 pages.
Cloth DM 136,—, öS 950,—
ISBN 3-211-81750-6

Contents:

Advances: R. J. S. Wise, G. L. Lenzi, and R. S. J. Frackowiak: Applications of Positron Emission Tomography to Neurosurgery. — J. Siegfried and T. Hood: Current Status of Functional Neurosurgery. — B. Pertuiset, D. Ancri, J. P. Sichez, M. Chauvin, E. Guilly, J. Metzger, D. Gardeur, and J. Y. Basset: Radical Surgery in Cerebral AVM — Tactical Procedures Based upon Hemodynamic Factors.

Technical Standards: M. Sindou and A. Goutelle. Surgical Posterior Rhizotomies for the Treatment of Pain. — A. Kumar and U. Fisch: The Infratemporal Fossa Approach for Lesions of the Skull Base.

Advances and Technical Standards in Neurosurgery

Volume 11

1984. 1 portrait. 80 figures. XII, 248 pages.
Cloth DM 139,—, öS 970,—, ISBN 3-211-81806-5

Contents:

Hugo Krayenbühl — An Appreciation (By M. G. Yaşargil)

Advances: G. M. Bydder: Nuclear Magnetic Resonance Imaging of the Central Nervous System — G. Huber and U. Piepgras: Update and Trends in Venous (VDSA) and Arterial (ADSA) Digital Subtraction Angiography in Neuroradiology.

Technical Standards: M. G. Yaşargil, L. Symon, and P. J. Teddy: Arteriovenous Malformations of the Spinal Cord — C. Lapras, R. Deruty, and Ph. Bret: Tumors of the Lateral Ventricles — F. Loew, B. Pertuiset, E. E. Chaumier, and H. Jaksche: Traumatic, Spontaneous and Postoperative CSF Rhinorrhea.

Volume 12

1985. 49 partly colored figures. XI, 186 pages.
Cloth DM 126,—, öS 880,—, ISBN 3-211-81877-4

Contents:

Advances: Valerie Walker and J. D. Pickard: Prostaglandins. Thromboxane, Leukotrienes and the Cerebral Circulation in Health and Disease.

Technical Standards: M. G. Yaşargil, P. J. Teddy, and P. Roth: Selective Amygdalo-Hippocampectomy. Operative Anatomy and Surgical Technique — E. Pásztor: Transoral Approach for Epidural Craniocervical Pathological Processes.

Volume 13

1986. 77 partly colored figures. IX, 179 pages.
Cloth DM 125,—, öS 870,—, ISBN 3-211-81885-5

Contents:

Advances: J. M. Tew Jr., and W. D. Tobler: Present Status of Lasers in Neurosurgery.

Technical Standards: H. G. Wieser: Selective Amygdalohippocampectomy: Indications, Investigative Technique and Results — F. Epstein: Spinal Cord Astrocytomas of Childhood.

Volume 14

1986. 71 partly colored figures. XIII, 230 pages.
Cloth DM 163,—, öS 1140,—, ISBN 3-211-81930-4

Contents:

Advances: H. B. Griffith: Endoneurosurgery: Endoscopic Intracranial Surgery — L. Symon, F. Momma, K. Schwerdtfeger, P. Bentivoglio, I. E. Costa e Silva, and A. Wang: Evoked Potential Monitoring in Neurosurgical Practice — K. von Werder: The Biological Role of Hypothalamic Hypophysiotropic Neuropeptides.

Technical Standards: D. Fohanno and A. Bitar: Sphenoidal Ridge Meningioma — H. J. Hoffmann, R. W. Griebel, and E. B. Hendrick: Congenital Spinal Cord Tumors in Children — Controversial Views of Editorial Board on the Intraoperative Management of Ruptured Saccular Aneurysms.

www.ingramcontent.com/pod-product-compliance
Lightning Source LLC
Chambersburg PA
CBHW071440230926
51846CB00001B/290
* 9 7 8 3 7 0 9 1 7 3 8 5 5 *